O N

OXFORD NEUROL

Stroke

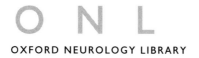

OXFORD NEUROLOGY LIBRARY

Stroke

Michael G. Hennerici
Rolf Kern
Kristina Szabo
Johannes Binder

Department of Neurology, University of Heidelberg,
Universitätsklinikum Mannheim, Mannheim, Germany

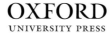

OXFORD
UNIVERSITY PRESS

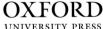

Great Clarendon Street, Oxford OX2 6DP,
United Kingdom

Oxford University Press is a department of the University of Oxford.
It furthers the University's objective of excellence in research, scholarship,
and education by publishing worldwide. Oxford is a registered trade mark of
Oxford University Press in the UK and in certain other countries

British Library Cataloguing in Publication Data

Data available

Library of Congress Cataloging in Publication Data

Data available

ISBN 978–0–19–958280–8 (paperback)

Printed in Great Britain
on acid-free paper by
Ashford Colour Press Ltd, Gosport, Hampshire

Contents

Section D **Secondary prevention, recovery and rehabilitation**

Preface

In the last decade the management of stroke patients and prevention of cerebrovascular diseases has become the most challenging task for neurologists, in particular in industrialized countries with an increasingly ageing population. Stroke is the most common cardiovascular disorder after heart disease with an estimated prevalence in Europe of nearly 10 million. It is also a major public health issue, very often causing immobility and long-term disability with enormous economic consequences. Although mortality has decreased significantly since the 1990s, many patients still suffer from permanent dependency despite increasing efforts to treat patients after acute onset in Stroke Units and Comprehensive Stroke Centres, which significantly improve the chances for full recovery and independence. This is in part due to increasing numbers of patients treated with thrombolysis for acute ischaemic stroke but also results from the interactive, multi-professional management of monitored intensive care through a primary care team according to a strict and evidenced-based operation procedure protocol. Adequate information among the public and health authorities about qualifying signs and symptoms of acute stroke victims are well established and the phrase "**Time is Brain and Stroke is an Emergency**" has been coined for health care strategies and public information in newspapers, television and advertisements. However, there are still limitations in knowledge, for example in transient ischaemic attacks being misinterpreted as a benign event, or stroke in the elderly with often delayed access to emergency admission on a Stroke Unit.

This small book is aimed at the multi-professional team on a Stroke Unit and early rehabilitation clinic as well as paramedics, and emergency and general physicians, who happen to see patients either very early after onset of stroke or after discharge from clinics. Chapters about appropriate diagnosis and treatment include updated knowledge about primary and secondary prevention and rehabilitation in patients who do not fully recover or develop cognitive impairment including vascular dementia.

This book provides information not only about ischaemic stroke—which represents the most common type of stroke caused by clot narrowing or blocking blood vessels (about 80%)—but also addresses haemorrhagic stroke caused from bleeding blood vessels in the brain or in the subarachnoid space (about 20%) including cerebral venous thrombosis, which is often overlooked (particularly in younger stroke victims). Diagnosis and diagnostic instruments as well as an aetiology-based new stroke sub-type classification based on evidence-based clinical phenomenology form an essential prerequisite for best management and specific treatment. There is also an update for secondary prevention including risk factor management with most recently developed and very promising anti-thrombotic agents, life-style modifications and evidence-based recommendations for interventional and medical treatment of stroke, risk factors and sources of embolism. Mechanisms of recovery and rehabilitation are now far better understood than they were ten or twenty years ago and offer a huge potential, in particular for those patients with focal disturbances of sensorimotor and neuropsychological deficits.

We have taken only a very limited number of references from a rapidly increasing number of exciting publications to attract the readers' interest for more learning either in a Stroke Unit team, through the internet, libraries, or during international stroke conferences.

All chapters have been written by current or previous members of the University of Heidelberg, Universitätsmedizin Mannheim, based on the expertise of a comprehensive Stroke Unit Centre founded there in 1998. We gratefully acknowledge the cooperation of our friends and colleagues and acknowledge their daily enthusiasm and dedication to treat more than 1000 stroke patients annually (up to 25% with thrombolysis), who teach us how to better meet their needs. We also gratefully acknowledge the cooperation of our colleagues in internal medicine, neuroradiology, neurosurgery, neuropsychology and radiology as well as our emergency and intensive care units for their support and the care of stroke patients. The chapter on stroke recovery was co-authored by V. Hömberg, an expert in treating patients after the acute phase in rehabilitation hospitals. Through the long-lasting experience and the interprofessional cooperation with our stroke nurses, behavioural therapists and physiotherapists, we have tried to prepare what we believe is a highly readable and extremely practical educational book to help readers in their own efforts to improve stroke care.

MG Hennerici, R Kern, K Szabo, and J Binder
Mannheim, July 2012

Foreword

MG Hennerici and colleagues have produced a welcome, compact and highly readable update on stroke.

The field is growing so rapidly it is (happily) proving difficult to keep book publications up to date. This publication focuses almost entirely on current concepts and is remarkably comprehensive for its page limits, including as well a thoroughly modern review of the literature.

It should prove helpful to those faced with problems in management and limited time for leisurely reading of the evolution of the concepts which currently drive modern clinical decisions.

JP Mohr
Daniel Sciarra Professor of Neurology
The New York Neurological Institute
December 2011

Abbreviations

ACA	anterior cerebral artery
ACE	angiotensin-converting enzyme
ADC	apparent diffusion coefficient
AF	atrial fibrillation
ANA	antinuclear antibody
aPL	antiphospholipid antibodies
ARB	angiotensin I/II receptor blockers
ASA	acetylsalicylic acid
ASL	arterial spin labelling
AVM	arteriovenous malformation
BA	basilar artery
BBB	blood brain barrier
bid	twice daily
CAA	cerebral amyloid angiopathy
CAD	coronary artery disease
CADASIL	cerebral autosomal dominant arteriopathy with subcortical infarcts and leukencephalopathy
CBF	cerebral blood flow
CNS	central nervous system
CRP	C-reactive protein
CSF	cerebrospinal fluid
CT	computed tomography
CTA	computed tomographic angiography
CVT	cerebral venous thrombosis
DSC	dynamic susceptibility contrast
DVT	deep venous thrombosis
DWI	diffusion-weighted imaging
ECG	echocardiogram
EVD	external ventricular drainage
GCS	Glasgow Coma Scale
HbA1c	haemoglobin A1c

HDL	high-density lipoprotein
ia	intra-arterial
ICA	internal carotid artery
ICH	intracerebral haemorrhage
ICP	intracranial pressure
im	intramuscular
INR	international normalized ratio
iv	intravenous
IVH	intraventricular haemorrhage
LDL	low-density lipoprotein
MCA	middle cerebral artery
MI	myocardial infarction
MRA	magnetic resonance angiogram
MRI	magnetic resonance imaging
NIHSS	National Institute of Health Stroke Scale
NINDS	Neurological Disorders and Stroke
NNT	number needed to treat
PAD	peripheral artery disease
PCA	posterior cerebral artery
PFO	patent foramen ovale
PTT	partial thrombin time
PWI	perfusion-weighted MRI
RCT	randomized clinical trials
RF	risk factor
SAH	subarachnoid haemorrhage
SVD	small vessel disease
SVE	subcortical vascular encephalopathy
TCD	transcranial Doppler ultrasound
TIA	transient ischaemic attack
tPA	tissue plasminogen activator
TTE/TEE	transthoracic/transoesophageal echocardiography
VA	vertebral artery

Epidemiology, pathophysiology and phenomenology

Chapter 1

Epidemiology

Key points

- Stroke is the third most common cause of death in industrialized countries and a major burden with increasing clinical, economic and social impact.
- Stroke is a growing issue of global health care due to the demographic development with increase of the elderly population. Due to a better management of risk factors and risk indicators (e.g. cardiovascular diseases) stroke mortality has decreased in the last 20yrs. However, morbidity is continuously increasing with age-related increase of atrial fibrillation and neurovascular degeneration (e.g. cerebral amyloid angiopathy-related intracranial bleedings).

3

1.1 Incidence and prevalence of stroke

Stroke is the most common cardiovascular disorder after heart disease, killing an estimated 5.7 million people annually worldwide (Figure 1.1). The prevalence of stroke in Europe has been estimated to be 9.6 million. Furthermore, stroke is a major public health issue and among the leading causes of immobility and long-term disability in developed countries. There are two main types of stroke. The most common is ischaemic stroke caused by clot narrowing or blocking of blood vessels (about 80%) followed by haemorrhagic stroke caused by a bleed from blood vessels in the brain or in the subarachnoid space (about 20%). With increasing age haemorrhagic stroke becomes more frequent and is estimated to grow within the next 10yrs up to 30%. Although mortality has decreased significantly, for many patients surviving can be worse than dying from stroke as severe disability is common and only about 40% receiving best medical treatment after acute onset in Stroke Units and Comprehensive Stroke Centres gain full recovery and independence. Stroke often results in widespread and long-lasting damage to patients' health causing weakness, paralysis or impairment of cognitive function

Fig 1.1 Global burden of stroke (source: WHO). See also Plate 1.

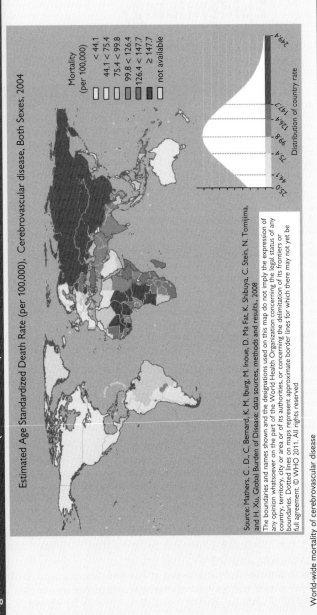

Estimated Age Standardized Death Rate (per 100,000), Cerebrovascular disease, Both Sexes, 2004

Mortality
(per 100,000)

< 44.1
44.1 < 75.4
75.4 < 99.8
99.8 < 126.4
126.4 < 147.7
≥ 147.7
not available

Distribution of country rate

Source: Mathers, C. D., C. Bernard, K. M. Iburg, M. Inoue, D. Ma Fat, K. Shibuya, C. Stein, N. Tomijima, and H. Xu, Global Burden of Disease: data sources, methods and results, 2008

World-wide mortality of cerebrovascular disease

including vascular dementia. World wide stroke leaves 5 million people permanently disabled. Stroke accounts for 2–3% of the total health care in the European Union with a calculated cost of €38 billion in 2006.

The onset of stroke is often sudden; about 25–30% of patients have immediate full recovery (TIA; transient ischaemic attacks), which despite increasing public awareness is still misinterpreted as a benign event. However, the risk of a permanent stroke after TIA is high (up to 20% within 4 weeks), in particular immediately after onset of first qualifying signs and symptoms, and in the presence of carotid or cardiogenic embolism. Thus, adequate information about the phenomenology and best management of patients is mandatory to prevent a severe and disabling stroke: the phrase 'Time is Brain and Stroke is an Emergency' has been coined for public information and health care strategies to improve current knowledge about the risks of stroke. This is not only important for the elderly. Stroke increasingly affects young adults aged 15–45yrs with a poor prognosis: 6yrs after stroke only 45% are still alive, and are not disabled or have not suffered from a recurrent vascular event.

1.2 **Risk factors for stroke**

Risk factors for stroke may be classified according to whether they are a) non-modifiable, b) well-documented and modifiable or c) less-well documented or potentially-modifiable (Table 1.1).

Hypertension is the most important risk factor for stroke: more than two-thirds of patients suffering a first stroke have elevated blood pressure (>130/80mmHg). An estimated 80% of the stroke burden attributable to hypertension and various cardiovascular endpoints occur in lower and middle social groups, and over 50% in patients >45yrs of age. Type 2 diabetes mellitus is linked to susceptibility of atherosclerosis and augments the atherosclerotic risk if hypertension, obesity and dyslipidaemia occur incidentally. Although type 1 diabetes mellitus elevates stroke risk, as well, it is often controlled and responds to improved management and treatment. With increasingly ageing populations type 2 diabetes becomes more frequent, and is often insufficiently managed because of poor compliance. Unfortunately, contradictory results have been reported from large randomized clinical trials (RCTs), finally suggesting that even best glucose control (HbA1-c ≤6), does not reduce the associated stroke risk at least in elderly patients. Dyslipidaemia has not been shown to contribute to stroke in general as a risk factor; however, it definitely is an important risk factor for coronary (CAD) and peripheral artery disease (PAD), and thus indirectly increases stroke risk. In addition, RCTs have shown that statins are beneficial and

Table 1.1 Risk factors for stroke

Non-modifiable risk factors
Age
Race
Sex
Family history
Genetic diseases, e. g.
　Moya-moya disease
　CADASIL, COL4A1, hereditary cavernous malformations

Well-documented and modifiable risk factors
Cardiovascular disease
　Coronary artery disease
　Non-valvular atrial fibrillation
Cerebral large artery disease
Cerebral small artery disease
Peripheral artery disease
Hypertension (>130/80mmHg)
Diabetes mellitus
Dyslipidaemia
　High total cholesterol
　High low-density lipoprotein cholesterol (>190mg/dL)
Environmental and social life-style factors
　Cigarette smoking
　Obesity, physical inactivity
Dietary factors
　Sodium intake >2.300mg
　Potassium intake <4.700mg
Arterial dissection
Arteritis/vasculitis
Sickle cell disease
Fabry disease

Less-well documented or potentially modifiable risk factors
Metabolic syndrome
Alcohol use (>5 drinks/day or more than moderate intake)
Hyperhomocysteinemia
Patent foramen ovale (PFO)
Drug abuse
Hypercoagulability
Oral contraceptive use
Acute/chronic inflammation (poor dental health care)
Migraine including genetic forms
High lipoprotein (a), high triglycerides, HDL cholesterol
High lipoprotein-associated phospholipase A_2
Sleep apnoea

significantly reduce the risk of secondary stroke in both patients with ischaemic and haemorrhagic causes, even if normal values of low-density lipoprotein (LDL, >100 <190mg/dL) are observed. Recommendations of the American Heart Association/American Stroke Association and European Stroke Organization concluded that lipid modifying drugs can reduce the risk of stroke both in persons with coronary heart disease and for secondary prevention of stroke even in the absence of co-existing coronary artery disease. Cigarette smoking is another key risk factor in particular for PAD and may increase stroke risk and mortality by about 1.5–2.0 times if associated with multi-vessel disease (cerebral artery disease, CAD and PAD). Smoking cessation may reduce the stroke risk after about 2yrs; and by 5yrs the level of risk reaches that of non-smokers.

1.3 **Cardiovascular disease**

Risk factors for stroke are often risk factors for other cardiovascular diseases, and atherosclerosis of cerebral arteries often coincides with CAD and PAD. The relative risk for stroke in patients with CAD is estimated to be 1.8 for men and 1.6 for women. In patients with significant large artery disease, coincidental CAD is common and increases with severity and number of cerebral arteries involved. This is also true for patients with PAD who share the highest morbidity and mortality because of frequently co-existing CAD and cerebral artery disease. Non-valvular atrial fibrillation (AF) is the most common sustained abnormal heart rhythm in adults and the major risk factor for stroke in an increasing ageing population. AF describes cases where rhythm disturbance is not associated with the problem of the mitral valve in the heart or rheumatic heart disease. In patients with AF the atria stop contracting because of rapid and irregular electrical impulses, which results in dilatation of the chamber walls and increasing thrombo-embolism from the left atrium after clot generation. Approximately 6 million individuals in Europe have AF and it is likely that this number will increase 2.5-fold by 2050 as a result of an ageing population, and improved survival of patients with cardiovascular conditions, which predispose to AF (Figure 1.2). The rate of death due to stroke is nearly 2-fold higher in men and 3-fold higher in women with AF compared with those without AF. Stroke as a result of AF is the most severe because of thrombo-embolism in large cerebral arteries leading to substantial territorial infarction with a high risk of secondary haemorrhagic transformation or parenchymal haemorrhage. Thus, the mortality and disability rates are high (up to 50% likelihood of death within 1yr). Co-existing major modifiable risk factors are common in people with AF and increase the likelihood of suffering from stroke

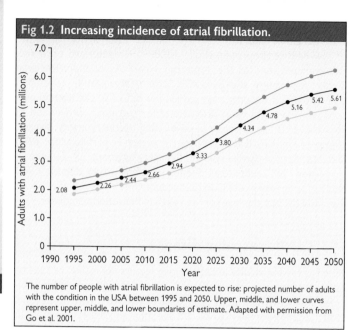

Fig 1.2 Increasing incidence of atrial fibrillation.

The number of people with atrial fibrillation is expected to rise: projected number of adults with the condition in the USA between 1995 and 2050. Upper, middle, and lower curves represent upper, middle, and lower boundaries of estimate. Adapted with permission from Go et al. 2001.

and vascular dementia based on different pathomechanisms becoming active in the same patient if not prevented by adequate lifestyle, management and risk factor treatment. High blood pressure is therefore responsible for a greater proportion of stroke, not only as a singular risk factor, but also as a co-factor for patients suffering from AF: AF confers a 5-fold increase in the risk of stroke compared with an approximately 3-fold risk of high blood pressure, and an 8-fold risk for those patients with AF who also have high blood pressure (Figure 1.3). Thus, a holistic approach to management is required. Vice-versa, the most common underlying causes of AF are increasing age and high blood pressure, and to a lesser extent ischaemic heart disease and diabetes. Dietary, lifestyle, and other factors, such as emotional and physical stress, and excessive caffeine, alcohol, or drug abuse have been identified as cofactors causing AF and stroke. In addition, there are also some data suggesting that the incidence of AF is higher than normal in athletes or people with increasing frequency of vigorous exercise (e.g. joggers)—thus, it is not just a condition of the elderly, but may occur in physically active younger people. Obesity and physical inactivity, as well as nutrition problems (e.g. potential effects of abnormal sodium and potassium intake on excessive variability of blood pressure regulation) are secondary risk factors for stroke with an estimated relative risk of 1.75–2.37. A sedentary lifestyle increases the risk of stroke by almost 3 times

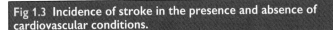

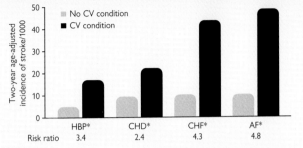

Fig 1.3 Incidence of stroke in the presence and absence of cardiovascular conditions.

AF, atrial fibrillation; CHD, coronary heart disease; CHF, congestive heart failure; HBR, high blood pressure

Two-year age-adjusted incidence of stroke in the presence and absence of cardiovascular (CV) conditions. Atrial fibrillation confers a fivefold increase in the risk of stroke; in patients with high blood pressure, stroke risk is increased threefold. *$p < 0.001$. Adapted with permission from Wolf et al. 1991.

and, hence, moderate physical activity is recommended to reduce the risk of stroke.

References

Go AS, Hylek EM, Phillips KA, et al. (2001) Prevalence of diagnosed atrial fibrillation in adults: national implications for rhythm management and stroke prevention: the AnTicoagulation and Risk Factors in Atrial Fibrillation (ATRIA) Study. *JAMA* **285,** 2370–5.

Truelsen T, Piechowski-Jozwiak B, Bonita R, et al. (2006) Stroke incidence and prevalence in Europe: a review of available data. *Eur J Neurol* **13,** 581–98.

Wolf PA, Abbott RD, Kannel WB. (1991) Atrial fibrillation as an independent risk factor for stroke: the Framingham Study. *Stroke* **22,** 983–8.

Chapter 2

Primary prevention

> ## Key points
> - The five major modifiable risk factors are high blood pressure, hyperlipidaemia, diabetes mellitus, cigarette smoking, and atrial fibrillation.
> - Modifiable risk factors should be treated and continuously monitored to prevent stroke, and reduce cardiovascular morbidity and mortality.
> - Urgent action is needed to prevent first and repeat stroke, in particular if transient ischaemic attacks (TIAs) occur. TIA patients with a high number of risk factors and risk indicators, and with early signs of brain ischaemia on magnetic resonance imaging (MRI) are at highest risk for early subsequent stroke.

Large artery disease, in particular in co-existing coronary artery (CAD) and peripheral artery diseases (PAD), is commonly associated with and caused by the aforementioned modifiable risk factors. They should be treated accordingly and controlled adequately (Table 2.1). Interventional or surgical treatment of patients with asymptomatic extracranial (in particular of the carotid arteries) or intracranial cerebral arteries is not recommended because of lacking evidence of substantial benefit to reduce the risk of stroke beyond best medical risk factor management.

Oral anticoagulation is recommended in most patients with atrial fibrillation (AF), whether permanent or paroxysmal. Adequate recognition and an increase in awareness of AF and AF-related stroke among the general public, patients, and health carers is mandatory. As new strategies for AF treatment and new anticoagulants become available in the near future, primary prevention is essential to reduce the burden of stroke in an increasingly ageing population (see Chapter 14).

Primary prevention also includes strong efforts to inform and update the public and medical community about warning signs for stroke and transient ischaemic attacks (TIAs) as well as a better understanding

Table 2.1 Scheme of the evidence and effectiveness of recommended actions in the primary prevention of stroke (modified from *Akt. Neurol.* 2010)

Type of intervention	Level of recommendation	Prevalence in the population	Rel. RR per year	Rel. RR per year	NNT	Remarks
Antihypertensive therapy	A	20–40%	30–40%	0.5%	20–100	Most important preventive action
Atrial fibrillation: anticoagulation	A	1%	59%	2.7%	37	Proven in high risk patients
Atrial fibrillation: antiplatelet therapy	B		29%	1.5%	67	In low or intermediate risk
Statin therapy in hypercholesterinaemia	A	5–10%	20%	1%	100	Only in high risk patients. Prevention mainly of atherosclerotic manifestations
Operation of asymptomatic carotid stenosis (>60% ACST)	A	5%	30–40%	0.5–1%	100–200	Only effective if the periprocedural risk is <3% in selected patients
Nicotine abstinence	B	20%	50%	?	?	Almost no elevated vascular risk after 10yrs
Weight normalization	B	20%	?	?	?	Multidimensional effect
Physical activity	B	–	25–48%	?	?	At least once a week
Antidiabetic therapy	C	3–5%	?	?	?	Reduction of stroke not convincingly documented

RR: risk reduction; NNT: number needed to treat

of early risk factors such as high blood pressure, hyperlipidaemia, diabetes mellitus, cigarette smoking, and lifestyle problems.

A careful history of the patients' potential risk factors including a specific family history for vascular diseases is as important as a detailed report about other factors forming a vascular risk profile and recent signs or symptoms of diseases in whatever vascular territory of the body. Additional investigations are: electrocardiogram (ECG), neurological and physical examinations, ultrasound studies of the extracranial and intracranial arteries, echo-cardiography, brain imaging and laboratory tests may follow depending on the aforementioned reports.

2.1 **High blood pressure**

As hypertension is the by far most important risk factor both for first stroke and stroke recurrence adequate diagnosis and treatment is of utmost importance. Many trials have shown the benefit of blood pressure control in all age groups and all degrees of hypertension.

A meta-analysis of multiple treatment trials showed that a 10-mmHg increase of systolic blood pressure increases stroke morbidity by 20% and mortality by 56%. The mean reduction in diastolic blood pressure of 5–6mmHg correlates with a 35–40% reduction in incidence of stroke. Treatment is valid in different races and ages, including the very old. Further studies showed that targeted blood pressure levels of 130/85mmHg reduce the risk of both ischaemic and haemorrhagic strokes in particular in patients with diabetes. While in a general population further lowering of blood pressure may still be better in an attempt to minimize the stroke risk associated with hypertension <130/80–85mmHg, RCTs have shown that this may result in an increasing rate of myocardial infarction and, hence, should be avoided, particularly in elderly subjects.

Although lowering blood pressure is clearly beneficial, the best drug and lifestyle regimen to achieve this is unclear. Many studies comparing the effects of diuretics, calcium channel antagonists, alpha- and beta blockers, angiotension-converting enzyme (ACE) inhibitors and angiotensin I/II receptor blockers (ARB) provided sufficient evidence for good blood pressure lowering. Additionally, beneficial effects beyond blood pressure lowering have been reported. The Anti-Hypertensive and -Lipid Lowering Treatment to Prevent Heart Attacks Trial (ALLHAT) showed that thiazide diuretics were more effective at reducing the risk of cardiovascular events than ACE inhibitors or alpha-blockers. The Heart Outcomes Prevention Evaluation (HOPE) trial showed that the ACE inhibitor ramipril reduced the risk of stroke and myocardial infarction, with a 0.68 relative risk for stroke ramipril vs. placebo. In addition, ACE inhibitors and ARBs may also have a beneficial effect on cardiovascular events and stroke beyond blood pressure lowering especially in patients with diabetes. In the 'Losartan Intervention For Endpoint reduction of hypertension (LIFE)' study, patients treated with losartan had a 24.9% relative risk reduction of stroke over the atenolol group.

A more recent meta-analysis among different anti-hypertensive drugs for the primary prevention of stroke in patients without CAD revealed a superiority of calcium antagonists, while beta-blockers were less effective than others. Although still recommended in patients with CAD, critical re-analysis of older trials have shown that, in patients with uncomplicated hypertension, beta-blockers failed to show protective effects compared with calcium channel antagonists, ARBs, or thiazide diuretics. Rather, they showed evidence of worse outcomes, particularly with regard to stroke. Thus, the available evidence does not support the use of beta-blockers as first-line drugs in the treatment of hypertension in general. Considerations for initial therapy should include thiazide diuretics, (with increasing dosages in patients with difficulties in controlling hypertension even if 3 or 4 drugs are used in combination), ACE inhibitors, calcium-channel blockers, ARBs alone or in combination, e.g. if ACE inhibitors and calcium channel blockers, and thiazide are present. ARBs should not be included unless compelling indications are present to suggest consideration of treatment in high risk patients with CAD or AF; in patients with cerebrovascular disease, an ACE inhibitor/diuretic combination is preferred as evidenced from one of the few secondary prevention studies in stroke patients (PROGRESS).

The European Society of Hypertension (ESH) risk chart (Figure 2.1) indicates an approximate risk of cardiovascular morbidity and

Fig 2.1 The European Society of Hypertension (ESH) risk chart.

	Blood pressure (mmHg)				
Other risk factors, OD or Disease	Normal SBP 120–129 or DBP 80–84	High normal SBP 130–139 or DBP 85–89	Grade 1 HT SBP 140–159 or DBP 90–99	Grade 2 HT SBP 160–179 or DBP 100–109	Grade 3 HT SBP ≥ 180 or DBP ≥ 110
No other risk factors	Average risk	Average risk	Low added risk	Moderate added risk	High added risk
1–2 risk factors	Low added risk	Low added risk	Moderate added risk	Moderate added risk	Very high added risk
3 or more risk factors, MS, OD or Diabetes	Moderate added risk	High added risk	High added risk	High added risk	Very high added risk
Established CV or renal disease	Very high added risk	Very high added risk	Very high added risk	Very high added risk	Very high added risk

The added absolute 10-year risk of fatal or non-fatal cardiovascular (CV) events as predicted by blood pressure, traditional CV risk factors, the metabolic syndrome (MS), subclinical CV organ damage (OD), diabetes and CV or renal disease. HT, hypertension; SBP, systolic blood pressure; DBP, diastolic blood pressure. Adapted from Mancia et al., 2007.

mortality in the following 10yrs in patients with different blood pressure levels and other risk factors. The key messages are:

- All definitions of hypertension are arbitrary because the risk of cardiovascular morbidity and mortality decreases continuously with decreasing blood pressure down to an optimal blood pressure level 120/70mmHg;
- As hypertension is only one of several interacting cardiovascular risk factors, the absolute cardiovascular risk depends on all risk factors
- Treatment indications and goals are determined by the absolute cardiovascular risk, such as risk factors, subclinical vascular manifestation and recent cardiovascular symptoms.

2.2 **Diabetes mellitus**

Although diabetes mellitus is a relevant and independent risk factor for stroke, only few studies reveal a significant reduction of stroke and other cardiovascular manifestation following strict anti-diabetic management. A 'healthy lifestyle' including diet, regular physical exercise, antidiabetic drugs or insulin if needed is as important as early management of vascular risk factors (e.g. hypertension, hyperlipidaemia) to prevent stroke.

The United Kingdom Prospective Diabetes Study (UKPDS) is the only completed large-scale primary prevention outcomes study to assess glucose control in type 2 diabetes. Intensive glucose control with insulin and/or sulphonylureas produced a non-significant 11% proportional increase in the risk of stroke relative to a less intensive lifestyle intervention. However, in a supplementary study of over-weight patients with type 2 diabetes, intensive therapy with metformin produced a non-significant 41% proportional reduction in the risk of stroke relative to lifestyle intervention. The effects of metformin on macrovascular outcomes may be independent (at least in part) of its ability to lower glucose. Nevertheless, a meta-analysis incorporating six randomized comparisons (three from the UKPDS and three from two small studies) showed a significant 42% incidence ratio reduction for stroke with intensive vs. less intensive glycaemic control strategies. On the other hand, the rate of non-fatal stroke was higher in patients treated aggressively to lower HbA1c values <6.0% in the recent ACCORD trial and there were no differences of stroke incidences between intensive and standard glycaemic control. The Emerging Risk Factor Collaboration study demonstrated based on data from 698782 people from 102 prospective studies that diabetes is a significant risk factor for ischaemic stroke (HR 2.27; [1.95–2.65]) and haemorrhagic stroke (HR 1.56 [1.19–2.05])

Fig 2.2 The predictive value of HbA1c and the risk for diabetes type 2, coronary heart disease (CHD), stroke and death

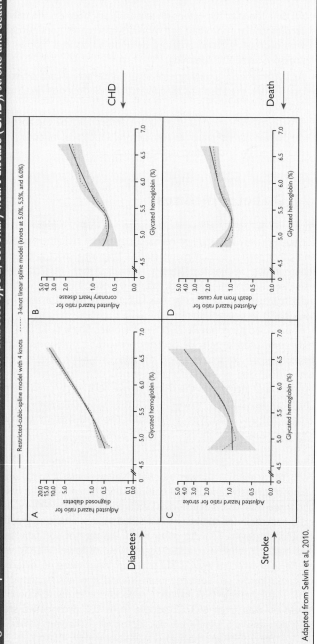

Adapted from Selvin et al, 2010.

as well as for all strokes (HR 2.27 [1.95–2.65]) and coronary heart disease (HR 2.00 [1.83–2.19]). Although HbA1c too is an important risk factor for stroke, cardiovascular disease and death with a significant predictive value (Fig. 2.2), the ACCORD trials failed to show that aggressive reduction of HbA1c levels (<6.0) vs. standard treatment (7–7.9%) reduced overall composite outcome–rather a higher mortality was observed (HR 1.19; 1.03–1.38 for death). Early and late follow-up (2008 and 2011) also failed to show significant macro- and microvascular benefits. This was in contrast to the UKPDS and DCCT studies, which suggested at least some benefits from intensive glycemic control with regard to nephropathy, retinopathy and small vessel disease of the brain. Final results from the ACCORD trial published in 2011 were very disappointing. This dilemma may be due to different study conditions and does not reflect real life at least in short-term trials: RCTs focus on particular inclusion and exclusion criteria and strategies exclusively addressing particular issues of interest (e.g. HbA1c control) in patients with longstanding atherosclerosis already fixed with a higher mortality rather than in pre-diabetic conditions with less severe arterial disease. Thus studies in patients with the metabolic syndrome at an earlier stage might be warranted in the future.

Treatment of co-existing hypertension and hyperlipidaemia, however, significantly lowers the risk of stroke in patients with type 2 diabetes. There is general consensus for treatment of hypertension in type 2 diabetes with the aim for a well-controlled systolic blood pressure of <130mmHg and, if possible, closer to lower values in this range, but not below 120mmHg, although the exact blood pressure goal has not been fully established. Furthermore, recent trials have shown that lipid-lowering therapy (mainly with statins, e.g. CARDS trial) significantly reduces primary stroke risk in patients with type 2 diabetes; benefit may even be apparent in those without markedly raised low-density lipoprotein (LDL) cholesterol levels.

2.3 **Hyperlipidaemia**

Although cholesterol as well as LDL cholesterol are by far less important as an individual risk factor for stroke than for CAD, only few studies have shown that statins can significantly reduce the risk of stroke in patients with previous strokes (i.e. the SPARCL trial). Many RCTs and meta-analysis have shown that statins reduce the risk of stroke in patients with elevated LDL cholesterol levels only. The JUPITER trial (Justification for the Use of Statins in Prevention: an Intervention Trial Evaluating Rosuvastatin) demonstrated that even in patients with normal LDL cholesterol values (<130mg/dL), but increased hs-C-reactive protein concentration (>2.0mg/L):

20mg rosuvastatin/day was better than placebo in reducing a combined outcome, including stroke and cardiovascular events. In a meta-analysis of more than 165,000 patients from 24 primary and secondary prevention trials a significant reduction of stroke could also be demonstrated. This effect is in part due to a reduction of elevated LDL cholesterol levels if more than 50% reduction can be achieved. However, it could also be observed in patients with normal LDL cholesterol values due to the modulating effect of statins for vasoprotective, anti-inflammatory, immunological, plaque stabilizing, and vasodilatatory responses, which have been suggested in RCTs similar to ARBs. Although details of action and the amount of benefit need further investigation, statins seem to postpone manifestation of type 2 diabetes rather convincingly and have been said to reduce the number of AF manifestation to some extent. There is no consensus about whether or not LDL cholesterol levels <70mg/dL are beneficial or may be harmful, especially in patients with previous intracerebral bleedings.

Thus, people with cholesterol levels >190mg/dL and/or cardiovascular disease including stroke/TIAs will most likely benefit from cholesterol-lowering regimens. They should definitely be treated continuously with statins. This recommendation is extended by more recent studies showing that aggressive treatment with statins in high risk patients is more effective than a moderate therapy (PROVE IT study, A- to -Z- study, TNT study).

Guidelines for primary prevention in hyperlipidaemia were summarized by the National Cholesterol Education Program (NCEP) Adult Treatment Panel III:

- Patients without CAD/0–1RFs should receive statins if LDL cholesterol is >160–190mg/dL
- Patients with ≥2RFs may be treated with statins if LDL cholesterol is >130–160mg/dL
- Patients with CAD should all be treated with statins, if LDL cholesterol is ≥70–100mg/dL.

2.4 **Cigarette smoking**

Many studies showed an increased risk of ischaemic stroke associated with smoking—in a meta-analysis of 22 studies cigarette smoking was found to be 1.92 (95% CI, 1.71–2.16). Ex-smokers tended to be at a lower risk than current smokers and in many studies ex-smokers did not reach statistical significance as an independent risk factor. This provides support that smokers can reduce their risk profile considerably by cessation of smoking. A possible mechanism for the increased risk of ischaemic stroke associated with smoking is that of accelerating large and small artery disease.

2.5 Alcohol consumption

A combination of deleterious and beneficial effects of alcohol is consistent with the observation of a dose relationship between alcohol and stroke. Elimination of heavy drinking can undoubtedly reduce the incidence of stroke. Otherwise, limited alcohol intake, preferably of red wine ('Bordeaux paradox'), may perhaps reduce the risk of stroke. However, it is unlikely that alcohol itself acts in a protective way, rather than particular substances, such as antioxidant and/or antiplatelet active components. Mechanisms of risks association are multiple and involve vascular as well as cardial sites (e.g. AF generation).

2.6 Lifestyle/obesity/physical activity

Dietary intake of fruit and vegetables ('Mediterranean cooking') reduces the risk of stroke, probably through antioxidant mechanisms or by raising potassium levels. Vitamin C, E, and beta-carotene belong to a group of free radical scavengers that are thought to act through the free radical oxidation of LDL cholesterol, which inhibits the formation of atherosclerotic plaques. The large Western Electric cohort found a moderate decrease in stroke risk associated with a higher intake of both beta-carotene and vitamin C. However, these data are insufficient to provide a sound evidence base for general recommendation. This is also true for other dietary factors associated with a small and inconsistently observed reduced risk of stroke, such as the consumption of low fat milk, calcium, fish oils, or black chocolate with a high concentration of cacao (>70%), which has more recently been claimed beneficial in reducing atherosclerosis and cardiovascular diseases.

Physical activity is of clear benefit in reducing the risk of heart disease and premature death. In combination with dietary factors it is one of the best strategies to reduce obesity and associated health problems, e.g. diabetes mellitus. Studies have also evaluated the association between physical activity and the risk of stroke, such as the Honolulu Heart Program, which investigated old and middle-aged men of Japanese ancestry. Other studies in patients at risk for stroke/TIA from small vessel disease have shown that physical activity is protective against development of lacunar strokes and white matter lesions and may be recommended also to decrease the likelihood of vascular dementia (see also results of the LADIS group). The protective effect of physical activity may be partly mediated through its role of controlling risk factors, such as hypertension, diabetes and obesity. Biological mechanisms such as increased HDL cholesterol and reduced homocysteine levels may also be responsible for the effect of physical activity.

So far none of the large studies addressing the potential impact of risk of hyperhomocysteinaemia for stroke have been able to demonstrate any significant general effects. Subgroup analysis of the recently presented VITATOPS study, however, gave some hints indicating that Vitamin B6, B12, and folic acid in patients with moderately to severely elevated hyperhomocysteinaemia (>17–18µmol/L) may be associated with risk reduction of stroke and vascular dementia attributed to small vessel disease. Unfortunately, the number of patients recruited into this sub-group was small as was the number of patients included for severe hyperhomocysteinaemia in this trial.

Hormone replacement therapy in post-menopausal women is associated with an increased risk of ischaemic stroke (HERS II trial) and should, therefore, not be used for primary prevention of stroke.

2.7 **Atrial fibrillation**

Atrial fibrillation (AF) is an epidemic affecting 1–1.5% of the population in the developed world. It is suspected to grow at least 3-fold by 2050. The health and economic burden imposed by AF and AF-related morbidity is enormous. AF has a complex mix of causes ranging from genetic to degenerative diseases, but hypertension and heart failure are the most common and epidemiologically most prevalent conditions. In addition, AF is often caused by myocardial infarction, mitral stenosis, thyrotoxicosis, alcohol, and often under recognized risk factors, such as obesity, metabolic syndrome, diastolic dysfunction, sleep apnoea, and psychological stress. AF is often undetected until a serious complication develops but may also last for decades without any complaints. Thus additional still unrecognized causes (e.g. inflammation or autoimmune mechanisms) may finally turn a harmless condition into a potentially serious source of embolism. Detection, diagnosis and monitoring of silent AF are therefore needed and routine pulse-taking plays an important role if public awareness in the detection of AF should be increased. Recently, the challenge of asymptomatic or silent AF has been recognized, and patients with undiagnosed AF may now receive better and easier preventive therapy. Strokes from AF are typically more severe and associated with greater disability. AF itself leads to more hospital admissions than any other arrhythmia.

A number of models have been devised to predict the risk of stroke and the likelihood of benefit from therapy with either warfarin or aspirin. Major risk factors were identified based on the pooled analysis of untreated patients from five primary prevention trials of warfarin (known as Atrial Fibrillation Investigator's risk stratification model, 1994) and the results from the aspirin arms of the Stroke Prevention in Atrial Fibrillation (SPAF I-III) studies. The CHADS2 score system was designed to simplify the determination of stroke risk in general practice and is widely used. This scheme is a mixture of five individual risk factors: congestive heart failure, hypertension, age >75yrs, diabetes mellitus, each of which is assigned 1 point, and prior stroke or TIA which is given 2 points. The stroke rate per 100 patient-years without anti-thrombotic therapy is expected to increase by a factor of 1.5 for each 1 point increase from 1.9 for a score of 0 to 18.2 for the highest score of 6. It has recently been extended to include vascular risk parameters (CHA2DS2-VASc-score: >75 yrs of age [2 points], vascular disease, age (65-74 yrs) and female gender [each assigned 1 point]).

Many RCTs have convincingly demonstrated the benefits of oral anticoagulation in patients with AF. Vitamin-K-antagonists, such as warfarin have consistently reduced the risk of ischaemic stroke or systemic embolism by about two-thirds compared with no treatment, and by 30–40% compared with aspirin in high risk patients with AF (Figure 2.3). However, treatment is underused for various reasons: the effect of warfarin is sensitive to changes in diet, liver function and drug interactions and, in particular, in old patients with cognitive deficits and repeat fall, compliance is limited. Thus, either a subtherapeutic international normalized ratio (INR) of 1.5–1.9 is used, which reduces the preventive efficacy of warfarin by a factor of 3.6 in patients <75yrs and by a factor of 2.0 in patients >75yrs when compared with the recommended INR values of 2.0–3.0. Although the risk of intracranial haemorrhage with controlled anticoagulation is small (0.3–0.5% per 100 patients-years) it increases exponentially to 2.7 per 100 patient-years at INR values between 4–4.5 and to 9.4% per 100 patient-years when an INR exceeds 4.5. Thus, a careful monitoring and co-operation of the patient is essential for a reasonable benefit to risk ratio.

New anticoagulants (oral thrombin antagonists or factor Xa inhibitors, e.g. dabigatran 110 or 150mg twice a day or rivaroxaban and apixaban) are on the horizon or have already been approved for

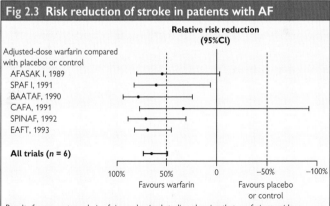

Fig 2.3 Risk reduction of stroke in patients with AF

Results from a meta-analysis of six randomized studies, showing that warfarin provides a greater reduction in the risk of stroke in patients with atrial fibrillation than does placebo. Adapted with permission from Hart et al. 2007. AF, atrial fibrillation; AFASAK I, AF, Aspirin, and Anticoagulation Study; SPAF I, Stoke Prevention in AF study; BAATAF, Boston Area Anticoagulation Trial for AF; CAFA, Canadian AF Anticoagulation Study; SPINAF, Stroke Prevention in Non-rheumatic AF; EAFT, European AF Trial.

patients with AF. They will considerably increase acceptance and reduce compliance problems because of a far easier management—in addition, there is preliminary evidence of an even better prevention of ischaemic stroke along with a reduced risk of intracerebral haemorrhage when compared with controlled warfarin INR 2.0–3.0 treatment (RE-LY, ROCKET and ARISTOTLE studies) (see Chapter 14).

Acetylsalicylic acid (ASA) is by far less effective than warfarin, although aspirin may reduce the risks of all strokes by approximately 20% compared with placebo. Even combinations of platelet anti-aggregating drugs did not show to be much better than aspirin alone. Aspirin was therefore recommended in patients with a lower or moderate risk of stroke and/or with contraindications to vitamin-K-antagonists. Again apixaban (5 mg bid) showed a significantly better benefit/risk ratio than aspirin (81–324 mg) (AVERROES).

However, patients diagnosed to have AF may also be treated with drugs or other strategies that control the abnormal heart rhythm itself. AF is commonly managed using 'rhythm control' or 'rate control' drugs—non-pharmacological methods to treat AF include electrical cardioversion and radio frequency catheter ablation, which is, at present, recommended in symptomatic patients with paroxysmal AF, rather than in asymptomatic patients or subjects with permanent AF. In the German AF ablation registry > 15,000 patients are listed: 70–85% were successfully treated, although repeat ablation had to be performed in 15–25% and mortality was 1.7% in a younger group <75yrs vs. 2.5% in those patients >75yrs old. More recently, and still experimental, percutaneous closure of the left atrial appendage was proposed in a first promising trial, which need confirmation in randomized series.

Current guidelines for the prevention of stroke in patients with AF are summarized in Table 2.2—they might be modified in the near future after recent approval of dabigatran, rivaroxaban and apixaban.

Table 2.2 European Stroke Organization guidelines for the primary prevention of stroke in patients with atrial fibrillation (level of evidence I/II, level of recommendation A)

Risk category	Current recommendation (2008)
Patients unable to receive anticoagulants	Aspirin (Class IA)
Patients <65yrs of age and free of vascular risk factors	Aspirin (Class IA)
Patients aged 65–75yrs and free of vascular risk factors	Aspirin or an oral anticoagulant (INR 2.0–3.0) (Class IA)
Patients aged >75yrs or who are younger with risk factors such as high blood pressure, left ventricular dysfunction or diabetes mellitus	Oral anticoagulant (INR 2.0–3.0) (Class IA)
INR, international normalized ratio.	

2.8 Patent foramen ovale and other cardioembolic sources

A patent foramen ovale (PFO) is an embryological remnant that may persist in some people (20–25%). Depending on the size of the PFO and its association with an atrial aneurysm, blood may be shunted from the right to the left atrium either spontaneously or during increased intrathoracic pressure (e.g. Valsalva manoeuvre). This may cause paradoxical embolism to the brain, e.g. in patients with acute venous thrombosis or co-existing hypercoagulable state, wherever present in the body. While some studies found PFO to be a stroke risk factor, in particular in younger patients, and if associated with convincing pathophysiological evidence causing a clot-dependent occlusion of an intracerebral artery, the risk of stroke in subjects with PFO in general is small. In a recent large study of >5000 patients less than 55yrs of age who suffered a stroke (SIFAP trial) the association with co-existing PFO was significantly higher than in a non-stroke population. Surprisingly, risk factors of atherosclerosis in young people were similar to the older population nowadays, which underlines the importance to generally manage and treat standard risk factors, rather than encourage interventional cardiologists to close PFOs. At present, there are no RCTs supporting anticoagulation or closure of PFO for primary prevention or in patients with stroke due to otherwise uncertain aetiologies apart from the presence of a PFO.

2.9 Asymptomatic stenosis of the internal carotid artery

The Asymptomatic Carotid Atherosclerosis Study (ACAS) and Asymptomatic Carotid Surgery Trial (ACST) included 1662 and 3120 patients respectively to study the efficacy and safety of carotid endarterectomy in primary prevention. The absolute risk reduction for stroke over a period of 5yrs was calculated as 5.4–5.9%, which equals an annual risk reduction of about 1% (number needed to treat, NNT = 100). This is about the same risk reduction which was achieved in patients with carotid disease in the SPARCL trial in symptomatic patients to prevent secondary stroke with 80 mg atorvastatin. According to both ACAS and ACST and meta-analyses the following sub-groups may probably benefit from carotid endarterectomy: men <65yrs, patients with a moderate stenosis >60–80% and with elevated serum cholesterol >250mg/dL, provided vascular surgeons applying for both studies were highly experienced and selected in order to achieve a very low complication rate (2.3% in ACAS and 2.8% ACST). Unfortunately, these figures cannot be taken for granted under non-trial conditions. Whether or not stenting is an alternative to surgery in this peculiar group of patients needs further careful studies: SPACE 2 is designed with three treatment arms to hopefully answer this question, whether surgery or stenting is better than best medical treatment alone. In CREST, 42.7% of patients had asymptomatic carotid disease: in contrast to previous trials the event rates were lower and ranged between 2.7% and 4.5% (4-year rates) CEA-group vs medical-therapy group (in ACST and ACAS 5-year rates ranged from 5.1–6.4% CEA- group vs. 11.0–11.8% medical-treated group). This marked reduction in event rates is impressive in particular in the medical-treated group, most likely due to better controlled management of risk factors of atherosclerosis in CREST and in general populations. CREST II is planned to test best medical therapy against CEA or CAS. Given these data and similar results from a subgroup of patients with carotid disease included in the SPARCL trial, which showed a significant reduction in event rates when treated with atorvastatin vs controls, best medical treatment with our without interventional approaches should be achieved.

2.10 Antithrombotic treatment for primary prevention

ASA is ineffective in primary prevention of stroke in males, however, in females >45yrs and with vascular risk factors ASA reduces the risk of stroke to a limited extent—bleeding risks may compensate this benefit. Other antiplatelet agents should not be used for primary prevention of stroke.

References

Amarenco P, Labreuche J. (2009) Lipid management in the prevention of stroke: review and updated meta-analysis of statins for stroke prevention. *Lancet Neurol* **8**, 453–63.

Brott TG, Hobson RW 2nd, Howard G, et al. (2010) Stenting versus endarterectomy for treatment of carotid-artery stenosis. *N Engl J Med* **363**, 11–23.

Connolly SJ, Ezekowitz MD, Yusuf S, et al. (2009) Dabigatran vs. warfarin in patients with atrial fibrillation. *N Engl J Med* **361**, 1139–51.

Connolly SJ, Eikelboom J, Joyner C, et al. (2011) Apixaban in patients with atrial fibrillation. *N Engl J Med* **364**, 806–17.

Diener HC, Aichner F, Bode C, et al. (2010) Primary and secondary prevention of cerebral ischemia. Joint Guidelines of the German Society of Neurology (DGN) and German Stroke Society (DSG). *Akt Neurol* **37**, e2–e22.

Everett BM, Glynn RJ, MacFadyen JG, Ridker PM. (2010) Rosuvastatin in the prevention of stroke among men and women with elevated levels of C-reactive protein: justification for the Use of Statins in Prevention: an Intervention Trial Evaluating Rosuvastatin (JUPITER). *Circulation* **121**, 143–50.

Furlan AJ, Reisman M, Massaro J, et al. (2012) Closure or medical therapy for cryptogenic stroke with patent foramen ovale. *N Engl J Med* **366**, 991–9.

Granger CB, Alexander JH, McMurray JJ, et al.; ARISTOTLE Committees and Investigators. (2011) Apixaban versus warfarin in patients with atrial fibrillation. *N Engl J Med* **365**, 981–92.

Hart RG, Pearce LA, Aguilar MI. (2007) Metaanalysis: antithrombotic therapy to prevent stroke in patients who have nonvalvular atrial fibrillation. *Ann Intern Med* **146**, 857–67.

Hennerici M, Aulich A, Sandmann W, Freund HJ. (1981) Incidence of asymptomatic extracranial arterial disease. *Stroke* **12**, 750–8.

Law MR, Morris JK, Wald NJ. (2009) Use of blood pressure lowering drugs in the prevention of cardiovascular disease: meta-analysis of 147 randomised trials in the context of expectations from prospective epidemiological studies. *Br Med J* **338**, b1665.

Lewington S, Clarke R, Qizilbash N, et al. (2002) Age-specific relevance of usual blood pressure to vascular mortality: a meta-analysis of individual data for one million adults in 61 prospective studies. *Lancet* **360**, 1903–13.

Mancia G, De Backer G, Dominiczak A, et al. (2007) ESH-ESC Guidelines for the management of arterial hypertension: the task force for the management of arterial hypertension of the European Society of Hypertension (ESH) and of the European Society of Cardiology (ESC). *J Blood Press* **16**, 135–232.

Patel MR, Mahaffey KW, Garg J, et al.; ROCKET AF Investigators. (2011) Rivaroxaban versus warfarin in nonvalvular atrial fibrillation. *N Engl J Med* **365**, 883–91.

PROGRESS Collaborative Group. (2001) Randomised trial of a perindopril-based blood-pressure-lowering regimen among 6,105 individuals with previous stroke or transient ischaemic attack. *Lancet* **358**, 1033–41.

Selvin E, Steffes MW, Zhu H, et al. (2010) Glycated hemoglobin, diabetes, and cardiovascular risk in nondiabetic adults. *N Engl J Med* **362**, 800–11.

Shinton R, Beevers G. (1989) Meta-analysis of relation between cigarette smoking and stroke. *Br Med J* **298**, 789–94.

Stone NJ, Bilek S, Rosenbaum S. (2005) Recent National Cholesterol Education Program Adult Treatment Panel III update: adjustments and options. *Am J Cardiol.* **96**, 53E–9E.

Chapter 3

Pathophysiology and cellular mechanisms

Key points

- Brain ischaemia initiates a cascade of events that evolve in time and space, and include harmful, as well as protective mechanisms.
- Many factors influence stroke development and final outcome such as: (1) individual time course and topography of brain ischaemia; (2) mechanisms active during impaired perfusion and reperfusion ('ischaemic core and penumbra'); (3) vascular collateralization and preserved integrity of neurovascular units and neuronal networks; and (4) neuronal repair strategies.
- Sequential neuroimaging (CT, MRI, ultrasound) supports the clinical diagnosis and monitoring of stroke victims, helps to identify complications, establish interventional treatment options and better predict prognosis

3.1 Cellular mechanisms

Brain ischaemia is caused by blockage of the vascular supply in the local region of the brain except when there is general circulatory failure due to cardiac arrest or systemic hypotension. Focal brain ischaemia typically results once a brain vessel has become occluded and causes a series of cellular and molecular events rapidly set in motion (Figure 3.1). In the centre ('ischaemic core') damage is severe and will be irreversible within minutes or hours leading to necrosis and death of neuronal, glial, and vascular cells ('ischaemic infarction'), unless rapid reperfusion occurs. The ischaemic core is surrounded by a less ischaemic area ('ischaemic penumbra') with neuronal tissue being temporarily inactivated, which may recover completely. However, as ischaemia persists, increasing components of the 'ischaemic penumbra' may also suffer the fate of the ischaemic core

Fig 3.1 Three phases of acute cerebral ischaemia induced damage, endogenous repair and regeneration (from Endres et al, 2008).

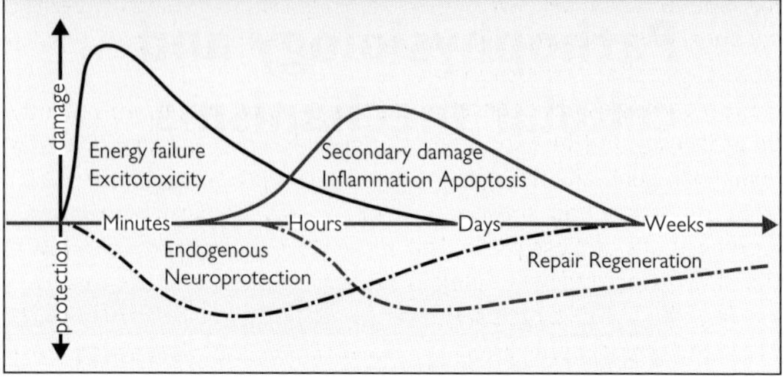

with functional impairment and necrosis. However, if the occluded artery reopens early and sufficient perfusion occurs with subsequent functional improvement or normalization of blood supply, the ischaemic lesion will remain limited and clinical deficits might well disappear ('transient ischaemic attack, TIA').

Focal cerebral ischaemia initiates a series of events ('ischaemic cascade'), which can lead to irreversible neuronal damage and cell death ('infarction'). The primary effects of ischaemia on brain tissue are reduced supply of substrate for energy metabolism (oxygen and glucose), depolarization of cells and swelling causing electrophysiological instability of the cell membrane, release of extracellular excitatory amino acids, efflux of K^+ ions and increased intracellular Ca^{2+} levels ('excitotoxicity phase'). Nitric oxygen (NO) derived from endothelial cells may increase blood flow, while neuronal and inducible NO synthase (NOS) contributes to the formation of peroxinitrite and hydroxyl anions. If the dramatic phase of early damage continues and the ischaemic core grows for many hours, secondary damage results from 'inflammation' and 'apoptosis'. Inflammation, although providing a necessary component for regeneration and repair, causes further lesion growth as does apoptosis, which may, however, also inhibit inflammation at a later stage. Thus, during the course of ischaemia similar biological mechanisms may be either deleterious or support repair and re-organization, which makes it difficult to recommend administration of pharmacological agents in patients that are beneficial under special circumstances, but potentially harmful at the same time. This 'Janus-faced' action of mechanisms might have been responsible at least to some extent for the obvious discrepancy between beneficial results reported from experimental stroke studies investigating particular components of action after selective treatment, who all failed in clinical trials eventually. This principle of both positive and negative action of drugs administered to treat stroke patients has also been confirmed from reperfusion studies using alteplase: once thrombolysis occurs, slow and incomplete recovery from oedema and cell swelling carries a high risk of neurotoxicity and secondary parenchymal intracerebral haemorrhage, in particular at later stages after onset of ischaemia.

New strategies have therefore been evaluated and, more recently, been investigated in experimental stroke beyond the only clinically approved agent (alteplase), e.g. GP IIb/IIIa receptor antagonists (SATIS trial) or ultrasound mediated thrombolysis ('sono-thrombolysis'). Combinations of these principles in 'low-dose' are suspected to lower the risks associated with alteplase, but increase the benefit eventually (e.g. the use of targeted abciximab research is microbubbles with local ultrasound administration). Further research is needed both experimentally and clinically to demonstrate whether the benefit-risk ratio of treatment using combined mechanisms in patients selected by refined imaging studies may lead to a wider application of thrombolytic agents ('imaging driven therapy'), for example, in extended or unknown time windows, ultra-early treatment with sequential strategies of combinations of thrombolytics and mechanical interventional devices ('bridging'), hypothermia, etc.

While thrombolysis is restricted to the first few hours after stroke, the utility of long-lasting current platelet aggregation inhibitors including GP IIb/IIIa receptor antagonists and anticoagulants, as well as antiplatelet agents is counterbalanced by the risk of intracerebral haemorrhagic complications. Novel strategies are based on better understanding of the molecular functions of different platelet receptors, such as glyco-protein Ib and VI: inhibition of these receptors in the mouse model prevented infarctions without increasing the risk of intracerebral bleeding. Furthermore, the intrinsic coagulation factors FXII and FXI play a functional role in thrombus stabilization during stroke: their deficiency or blockade in otherwise healthy subjects protects from cerebral ischaemia without obviously affecting haemostasis. Stroke patients may eventually benefit from such agents without the hazard of severe bleeding complications.

Our current pathophysiological understanding of stroke is based on the concept of an early ischaemic core, which is surrounded by the ischaemic penumbra with milder insults. In both highly vulnerable, rapidly changing and developing areas excitotoxic and inflammatory mechanisms may lead to cell death and apoptosis, but also protective programs of the brain are simultaneously active and important for good repair and recovery (Figure 3.2).

Most interestingly, ischaemia does not only affect the brain, but also extracranial systems inducing important immunosuppression via activation of the sympathetic nervous system in the body—from this bacterial infection can result, which is regularly seen in many stroke

Fig 3.2 Damaging and repair mechanisms at the neuro-vascular unit.

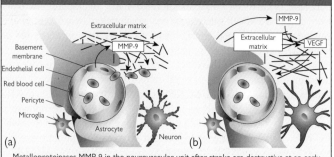

Metalloproteinases MMP-9 in the neurovascular unit after stroke are destructive at an early stage (opening of the BBB, causing apoptosis and secondary haemorrhage) (a), but are important for good repair at a later stage activating VEGF (b). Adapted from Zlokovic 2006.

Fig 3.3 Outcome after stroke under prophylectic antibiotic therapy.

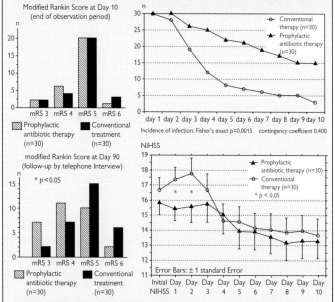

Outcome (mRS) after stroke under conventional treatment and prophylactic antibiotic therapy at end of study and 90 days after conventional treatment or prophylactic antibiotic therapy (mRS 0 = no symptoms, mRS 6 = death). The incidence of infection throughout the observation period was lower in the treatment group. At the end of the observation period, the outcomes were not different (NIHSS and mRS), but on follow-up at day 90, outcome was significantly better in the treatment group. Schwarz et al. 2008.

victims and probably should be prevented very early by adequate administration of antibiotics already prior to clinical signs of pulmonary or bladder infections. Several clinical and experimental studies have indeed shown that inflammation and infection contributing to a poor outcome and significantly higher mortality after stroke could be limited (Figure 3.3).

3.2 **The neurovascular unit**

The 'neurovascular unit (NVU)' in the setting of acute ischaemic stroke is a novel way to explore pathophysiological mechanisms, where the simultaneous interplay between microvessels (endothelial cells–basal laminar matrix–astrocyte end-feet), astrocytes, neurons and their axons, in addition to other supporting cells (e.g. microglia and oligodendroglia) is taken into account (Figure 3.2). The vulnerability and lack of protection of essential components of this neurovascular unit could partly explain the failure so far of clinical trials and neuroprotectants in acute stroke. The mechanisms and importance of the NVU to reductions of flow or to flow-cessation is unclear, but is likely to be complex beyond the individual component as they are connected through microvessels and dendritic connections. Thus, alterations in microvessel integrity could have effects on adjacent NVUs with impact on neuronal function and vice-versa. The simultaneous co-expression of matrix proteases by neurovascular cells and neurons and the responses of treatment targets to these specific agents in pre-clinical stroke/hypoxia models and in clinical trials is an important issue for future strategies to improve early management of acute stroke patients. Matrix–matrix receptor interactions with cerebral microvessels and the rapid expression of matrix-sensitive proteases during ischaemia and during repair in a later stage could be an important step not only in our understanding of the microvessel-neurocommunication, but also in future modelling of treatment strategies.

3.3 **Stroke recovery**

Within hours after onset of symptoms, a time-limited window of neuroplasticity opens during which the greatest gains in recovery occur. Plasticity mechanisms include activity-dependant rewiring and synapse strengthening, but also new learning in adjacent or remote neuronal networks. Neuroimaging significantly supports new strategies to improve stroke recovery and our understanding of how to optimally manage and modify surviving neuronal networks (for further details see Chapter 15).

3.4 **Imaging the pathophysiology of ischaemia**

Extra- and intracranial large artery disease, cardio-embolism and small vessel disease are the three leading causes of cerebral ischaemia. There are many other less common potential causes, which should be identified if possible. However, best medical work-up still results in about one-third of strokes remaining etiologically undiagnosed in the individual patient. It is well known, that stroke victims with particular sources of embolism are at high risk to suffer repeat ischaemic events, but one should bear in mind that a second stroke should not necessarily result from the same cause as the first event. It has not been common wisdom, that a multiplicity of stroke mechanisms (i.e. extensive risk-factors of atherosclerosis, large and small vessel disease) are also common in younger subjects suffering acute ischaemic strokes (<55yrs) likewise in an elderly population (>65yrs of age), whereas cardiogenic sources (e.g. non-valvular atrial fibrillation), small vessel disease (SVD) or cerebral amyloid angiopathy (CAA) definitely increase with age.

Multi-model imaging techniques such as computed tomography (CT), magnetic resonance imaging (MRI), and ultrasound (US) incorporating parenchymal depictions, illustration of the vasculature, and tissue perfusion data can provide a lot of information regarding the individual ischaemic pathophysiology. The information provided by modern neuroimaging precisely supports the clinician's interpretation about the topography of the clinical syndrome and symptoms, allows a better risk/benefit estimate as well as a refined selection of the best medical treatment for the individual patient. CT, MRI and US all provide slightly different information depending on the technical capabilities. In addition, they provide further insight into many active mechanisms, potential risks and compensatory strategies as well as for an adjusted evaluation of the prognosis in different phases of stroke development including a better follow-up once revascularization or complications occur.

Obstruction of the cerebral circulation is typically the initial event and the most obvious feature of cerebral ischaemia. It can be caused by partial or subtotal stenosis of extra- and intracranial large arteries, or alternatively, complete blockage of the vessel lumen, either from artery-to-artery embolism or local thrombosis. Vessel occlusion may be compensated in the presence of sufficient collateral circulation and tissue perfusion, which are individually quite heterogeneous. Refined techniques improving vascular imaging such as transcranial Doppler ultrasound (TCD) and angiographic techniques (computed tomography angiography, CTA, and magnetic resonance angiography, MRA) have contributed to a better understanding of active mechanisms and may play an important role in their diagnosis and management. Non-invasive imaging of collateral flow patterns in large cerebral arteries (e.g. at the Circle of Willis) has replaced conventional angiography today. Cerebral perfusion studies (CT perfusion, perfusion MRI, ultrasound perfusion imaging) are also useful to follow the recruitment of small vessels, capillary networks and venous outflow, which are important prognostic measures because of changing intraluminal pressure gradients and insufficient cerebrovascular autoregulation. These processes can be followed from the first hours after stroke onset until chronic stages of ischaemia and may become important in the future for our understanding of 'vascular dementia', which seems to be of much more complex nature (involving neurodegenerative and ageing processes) than hitherto assumed.

References

Endres M, Engelhardt B, Koistinaho J, et al. (2008) Improving outcome after stroke: overcoming the translational roadblock. *Cerebrovasc Dis* **25**, 268–78.

Schwarz S, Al-Shajlawi F, Sick C, Meairs S, Hennerici MG. (2008) Effects of prophylactic antibiotic therapy with mezlocillin plus sulbactam on the incidence and height of fever after severe acute ischaemic stroke: the Mannheim infection in stroke study (MISS). *Stroke* **39**, 1220–7.

Siebler M, Hennerici MG, Schneider D. et al. (2011) Safety of tirofiban in acute ischemic stroke: the SATIS trial. *Stroke* **42**, 2388–92.

Stoll G, Kleinschnitz C, Nieswandt B. (2008) Molecular mechanisms of thrombus formation in ischaemic stroke: novel insights and targets for treatment. *Blood*. **112**, 3555–62.

Zlokovic BV. (2006) Remodeling after stroke. *Nature Med* **12**, 390–1.

Chapter 4

Phenomenology of ischaemic stroke

Key points

- A transient ischaemic attack is not a benign disease but associated with a high risk of early recurrent stroke. 'TIA' patients with neurological symptoms lasting between 1 and 24hr often have ischaemic lesions on brain imaging.

- Common causes of ischaemic stroke in the elderly population are large artery atherosclerosis and cardio-embolism, leading to territorial and borderzone infarction, and small vessel disease being responsible for lacunar infarction and associated progressive neurological dysfunction (subcortical vascular encephalopathy).

- Other and rare causes need to be considered particularly in younger patients, such as inflammatory and non-inflammatory vasculopathies and coagulation disorders. However, strokes at younger age are more often associated with common vascular risk factors than hitherto assumed.

- Spinovascular disease is rare compared with cerebrovascular disease. The common causes of spinal cord infarcts are aortic disease or surgical procedures at the aortic level, small vessel disease including inflammatory vasculopathies, spinal or segmental artery compression or occlusion, severe hypotension and spinal cord AVM.

4.1 **TIA/acute cerebrovascular syndrome**

The original definition of a 'transient ischaemic attack' (TIA) suggested that such an event does not cause major harm to the brain but should be considered a warning sign in patients at risk to suffer from subsequent stroke. It describes the sudden occurrence of reversible neurological symptoms of presumed vascular aetiology limited to a maximum of 24hr. Several studies have shown, however, that the majority of 'TIA' patients with symptoms lasting more than 2hr have ischaemic lesions on brain imaging. Nowadays, patients should be treated within hours after the onset of ischaemic signs and/or symptoms with alteplase in particular if symptoms are fluctuating: the 'retrospective' definition of a TIA after 24hr is useless under such circumstances. This is why more recent proposals suggested to change the definition of a TIA in favour of a reduced time limit to 1hr or to use another terminology, i.e. 'acute cerebrovascular syndrome', which might be more appropriate for the acute setting. Using the term TIA, however, may still be justified in clinical trials where a *posteriori* diagnosis is possible and important to compare such trials with previous ones, which had used the old definition criteria.

TIA patients have a considerable risk of recurrent stroke, particularly early after the event (10–20% during the first 2 weeks, 3.7% per year). Approximately, 17% of TIA patients will not be able to carry out their activities of daily life 6 months after the event due to early stroke recurrence. Patients with longer TIA symptom duration, motor symptoms and/or speech disturbances and of older age have a higher risk of stroke. The risk of recurrent stroke may be estimated using the ABCD2 score with sum scores of ≥4 indicating a high risk of a stroke within 7 days (see Table 4.1).

It is very important in daily practise to identify the underlying cause of the ischaemic event and to initiate early secondary prevention. Apart from clinical characteristics individual patients are at highest risk with fluctuating symptoms often associated with active sources of embolism:

• Carotid disease (stroke risk more than 20% at 90 days)
• Cardiac source of embolism (e.g. 18-fold higher risk in atrial fibrillation [AF])

The identification of such conditions and subsequent early intervention are associated with a better outcome. All these high-risk patients should be admitted to a stroke unit within 24hr after onset of signs/symptoms irrespective of partial or full recovery within this time period.

Table 4.1 ABCD2 score for the risk assessment after TIA

Factor	Score
Age ≥60	1
Blood pressure ≥ 140/90mmHg at initial evaluation	1
Diabetes mellitus in patient's history	1
Symptoms:	
− Unilateral weakness	2
− Speech disturbance without weakness	1
− Neither	0
Duration of Symptoms	
− More than 60min	2
− 10–59min	1
− Less than 10min	0

4.2 Cerebral ischaemic stroke

4.2.1 Extra- and intracranial large artery disease

Large artery disease is the presumed cause of cerebral infarcts in 15–40% of patients, and in 10–15% of all patients admitted to stroke units for acute cerebrovascular events, a severe stenosis, or occlusion of the internal carotid artery (ICA) can be found (Figure 4.1). Atherosclerosis is the underlying disease related to this condition. The principal sites for atherosclerotic plaques are located in the ICA at the extracranial bifurcation or at the carotid siphon, and in the large intracranial arteries. Intracranial artery disease is less common in Western countries, and is more often diagnosed in Asian and black people. In the posterior circulation atherosclerotic lesions occur in the proximal and distal part of the vertebral arteries and in the basilar artery.

Besides the carotid and the vertebrobasilar systems, other potential sources of cerebral emboli include ulcerated plaques in the aortic arch and branching off arteries, such as the ostium of the left subclavian, the innominate and the left common carotid arteries; these have all been identified as responsible for a substantial proportion of strokes that occur in the absence of other known causes (Figure 4.2).

Fig 4.1 Stroke in ICA stenosis (see also Plate 2).

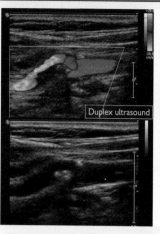
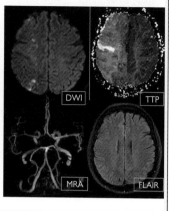

Proximal right ICA stenosis diagnosed by extracranial duplex ultrasound (left) with subsequent embolic infarction and extensive hypoperfusion (DWI and PWI, upper right) in the corresponding MCA territory.

38

The atheromatous plaque is characterized histologically by five factors:

- Increase in cholesterol
- Increase in connective tissue elements, especially elastins and glycosaminoglycans
- Smooth muscle cell proliferation
- Presence of foam cells (lipid-laden macrophages)
- Presence of inflammatory cells.

Different stages of development usually coincide in the same atheroma (Figure 4.3). Atherosclerosis is recognized as a disorder characterized by a chronic inflammatory dysfunction; key markers of acute inflammation and the innate immune response have been linked to the occurrence of myocardial infarction and stroke.

Atherothrombotic plaques often grow until total occlusion of the arterial lumen occurs without causing clinical signs or symptoms, provided that collateral blood flow capacities are maintained e.g. through anastomoses with the external carotid arteries and within the circle of Willis. Nevertheless, haemodynamic compromise may lead to the development of local embolism and cause—even years after vessel occlusion—downstream embolization in slow flow territories. This is especially common in 'borderzones' of the large cerebral arteries (Figures 4.4 and 4.5). Borderzone infarcts are common in significant large artery disease and may be linked

Fig 4.2 Predominant localization of atherosclerotic lesions of brain supplying arteries.

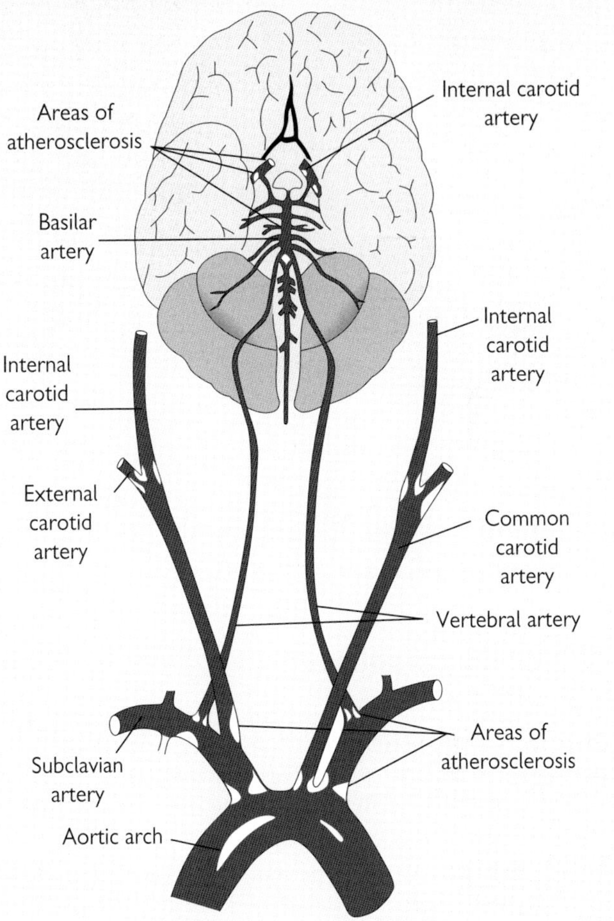

to impaired washout of micro-emboli lodged in the watershed areas.

On the other hand, plaque rupture and acute intraluminal thrombus formation with propagating emboli may turn a recent small silent plaque into a vulnerable plaque, which may obstruct small distal arteries in the brain causing territorial infarction. The embolic material can come from fibrin–platelet aggregations or from a red thrombus that occludes the extracranial artery.

Fig 4.3 The cascade of atherosclerosis.

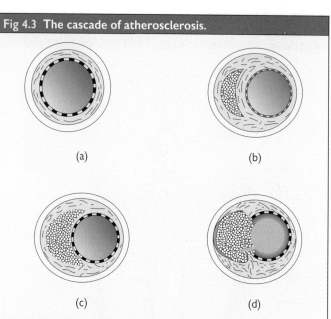

(a)

(b)

(c)

(d)

The cascade of atherosclerosis. (a) Normal artery, (b) early atheroma with a normal fibrous cap, (c) vulnerable plaque with a thin fibrous cap, large lipid pool and many inflammatory cells, and (d) plaque rupture and vessel thrombosis.

4.3 **Cardio-embolism**

Cardio-embolism is the presumed cause of cortical or large subcortical (e.g. lentiform nucleus) cerebral infarct in at least 15–30% of stroke patients (Figure 4.6), although definitive proof of embolization from the heart is often lacking. The most common potential

Fig 4.4 Cortical and subcortical borderzones of the cerebral arteries.

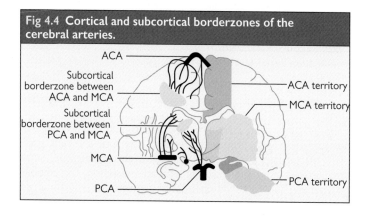

ACA

Subcortical borderzone between ACA and MCA

Subcortical borderzone between PCA and MCA

MCA

PCA

ACA territory

MCA territory

PCA territory

Fig 4.5 Borderzone infarction on MRI.

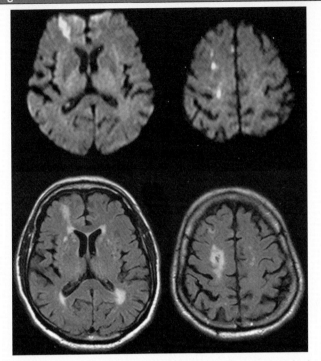

DWI (upper row) and FLAIR images (bottom row) of acute ischaemic lesions located in the right anterior cortical and the internal borderzone.

cardiac sources of embolism include dysrhythmias (e.g. AF or sick sinus syndrome) and structural changes (e.g. rheumatic heart disease, acute myocardial infarction, left ventricular akinetic segment or aneurysm, dilated cardiomyopathy, or prosthetic cardiac valves). Less common or less often detected sources are endocarditis and cardiac tumours. Paradoxical embolism via a patent foramen ovale has also been linked to stroke in young people (<55yrs), especially with the association of atrial septal aneurysm and deep vein thrombus (see Table 4.2).

With increasing age, cardio-embolism occurs more frequently as potential source of stroke, because AF becomes more prevalent. However, other potential sources are also increasing in an ageing population, e.g. small vessel disease and cerebral amyloid angiopathy: thus the presence of AF in a stroke patient does not justify an immediate diagnosis of a cardiogenic etiology unless further careful neuroimaging studies have been performed.

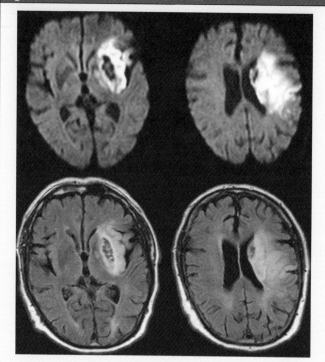

Fig 4.6 Cardioembolic stroke on MRI.

DWI (upper row) and FLAIR images (bottom row) of acute cardioembolic stroke located in the left MCA territory. Note significant haemorrhagic transformation in the lentiform nucleus often seen to result from recanalization of cerebral embolism.

4.4 Small vessel disease (micro-angiopathy)

Small vessel disease (SVD) accounts for about 15–40% of cerebral infarcts. It corresponds to *in situ* stenosis and occlusion of deep perforating branches of the hemisphere, and brainstem when atherosclerosis involves these small cerebral arteries, especially in patients with risk factors, such as hypertension and diabetes. In contrast to pial arterial branches, these perforators lack significant anastomoses, so there is no collateral supply when occlusion develops. Occlusion therefore leads to a small (lacunar) infarct limited to the territory of the occluded perforator (Figure 4.7). Radiologically, lacunes are defined as small deep lesions on brain imaging, usually less than 1.5cm in diameter with a density or signal consistent with an infarct in the appropriate area of the brain. In the absence of a responsible lesion on CT, magnetic resonance diffusion-weighted imaging (MR-DWI) often identifies these lesions. However, if investigations are delayed some lacunes go undetected. The small infarcts widely

Table 4.2 Common findings associated with cardio-embolism	
Rhythm disturbances	*Heart failure and cardiomyopathy*
– Atrial fibrillation	*Cardiac procedures*
– Atrial flutter	– Coronary artery bypass grafting
– Sick sinus syndrome	– Cardiac catheterization
Valvular heart disease	– Cardiac valve surgery
– Prosthetic valves	*Cardiac tumours*
– Rheumatic mitral stenosis	– Atrial myxoma
– Mitral valve prolaps	– Metastasis
– Calcific aortic stenosis	*Other (TEE findings)*
– Mitral annular calcification	– Patent formen ovale
Endocarditis	– Atrial septal aneurysm
Myocardial infarction	– Left atrial thrombus
– Acute	– Spontaneous echo contrast
– Chronic (regional dyskinesia)	

scattered throughout the deep white matter, might accumulate gradually. Each infarct may be inconspicuous, but their cumulative effect, together with deep white matter lesions—being also characteristic for SVD—is devastating with various neurological deficits, gait disturbances, urinary incontinence, and progressive cognitive decline (subcortical vascular encephalopathy, SVE). If associated with cardiac and kidney SVD, the prognosis of these patients is poor due to a high 5 year mortality (30–50%) (LADIS 2011).

4.5 **Mixed aetiologies and rare causes**

Between 5 and 25% of patients may have more than one of these three leading causes of stroke, and it may be difficult to determine their precise aetiology. Other potential causes become important in younger patients (≤45yrs). The main similarity between stroke in younger people and stroke in older people (>75yrs) is the importance of large artery atheroma and small vessel disease; cardio-embolic sources are less prominent and different in etiology (AF in the elderly, PFO in the younger stroke populations). This has been shown in contrast to what was commonly suspected by more recent studies (i.e. the SIFAP trial) investigating more than 5000 younger stroke patients. SIFAP demonstrated that the risk profile of atherosclerosis is more often responsible for stroke in the young than has hitherto been assumed.

Fig 4.7 Lacunar infarction on MRI.

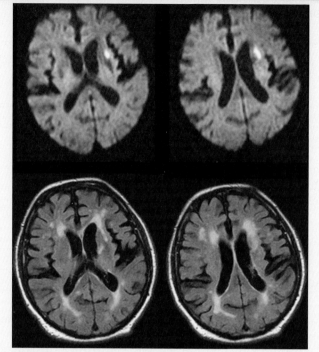

DWI (upper row) and FLAIR images (bottom row) of acute lacunar infarction located in the left putamen and associated with small vessel disease.

The aetiology cannot be determined in about 30% of patients, and these are termed cryptogenic strokes. This is particularly common if the TOAST criteria are used, which underestimate the high number of patients with SVD and falsely classify patients with multiple, coexisting causes of stroke as 'unidentified'. The more recently proposed ASCO classification should therefore be used preferentially not only for randomized trials, but also for clinical practise (see Chapter 9).

Less common causes of stroke (see Table 4.3) need explicit work-up: haematological abnormalities and coagulopathies are associated with an increased risk of ischaemic stroke. Polycythaemia (defined as a haematocrit above 0.50 in males and 0.47 in females) is associated with an increased risk of stroke, possibly from hyperviscosity of the blood or increased platelet activity causing thrombosis.

Antiphospholipid antibodies (aPL) are found in a variety of autoimmune disorders other than systemic lupus erythematosus, including rheumatoid arthritis, primary Sjogren's syndrome, progressive systemic sclerosis and Takayasu arteritis. These can accompany

Table 4.3 Summary of stroke aetiologies including rare causes

Embolism

Cardio-embolism

– Valvular abnormalities, e.g. mitral prolapse, endocarditis

– Myocardial hypokinesis

– Intracardial masses, e.g. atrial myxoma, sarcoma

– Atrial septal aneurysm

Paradoxic embolism

– Patent foramen ovale, atrial septal defect with right-to-left shunt

Non-cardiac embolism

– Pulmonary origin, e.g. pulmonary venous thrombosis, pulmonary AVM

– Arterial origin, e.g. aneurysm, dissection, vascular malformation

– Miscellaneous, e.g. fat, tumour, air

– Complications of neck and thoracic surgery

Vasculopathies

– Infectious, e.g. syphilis, tuberculosis, mycoplasma, HIV

– Inflammatory non-infectious, e.g. systemic lupus erythematodes, polyarteritis nodosa, temporal arteritis, Takayasu's disease, Wegener granulomatosis, Churg–Strauss syndrome, neurosarcoidosis, granulomatous angiitis of the CNS

– Vasospasm/vasoconstriction, e.g. migraine, drug-induced, catheter angiography, subarachnoid haemorrhage

– Congenital connective tissue disorders, e.g. Marfan's disease, Ehlers-Danlos syndrome, Fabry's disease

– Other non-inflammatory arteriopathies, e.g. fibromuscular dysplasia, Moya-moya disease, amyloid angiopathy, Sneddon's syndrome

Coagulopathies and haematological abnormalities

– Anaemia

– Immune-mediated, e.g. thrombotic thrombocytopenic purpura, antiphospholipid antibodies

– Hyperviscosity, e.g. sickle cell disease, thalassaemia, polycythemia vera, multiple myeloma, thrombocythemia

– Coagulation abnormalities, e.g. antithrombin III, protein C, protein S deficiency, factor V Leiden, prothrombin 20210 mutation, platelet hyperaggregability, disseminated intravascular coagulation, vitamin K therapy, oral contraceptives, paraneoplastic coagulation disorder

(continued)

Table 4.3 (Cont'd) Summary of stroke aetiologies including rare causes

Miscellaneous

- Trauma or mechanical arterial compression

- Cerebral venous thrombosis

- Increased intracranial pressure

- Mitochondrial disease, i.e. MELAS (mitochondrial encephalomyopathy, lactate acidosis, and stroke-like episodes)

- Cerebral autosomal dominant arteriopathy with subcortical infarcts and leukoencephalopathy (CADASIL)

malignancy, haematological disorders, such as idiopathic thrombocytopenic purpura, haemolytic anaemia or infections including syphilis, infection with human immunodeficiency virus and a variety of viral infections. Numerous studies have clearly shown an association between aPL and cerebral ischaemia. In general, stroke associated with aPL tends to occur in a younger population and there seems to be a slightly higher incidence in women.

Many case reports and case-control studies have been published related to the association of other coagulation abnormalities and stroke (e.g. factor V Leiden, prothrombin 20210 mutation, protein C deficiency, protein S deficiency, and antithrombin III deficiency). However, there have been no definitive conclusions. A number of prospective studies have also shown a strong association between elevated fibrinogen levels and risk for cerebral infarction.

Hyperaggregable platelets lead to intracranial thrombosis in thrombotic thrombocytopenic purpura, which can also result in intracranial haemorrhage when platelets are depleted. Sickle cell disease is associated with both intracranial and extracranial vasculopathy caused by inspissation of the sickle cells in the arterial wall resulting in thrombosis. Blood transfusion reduces the risk of stroke in children with sickle cell anaemia who have abnormal results on TCD.

Inflammatory vasculitis outside the brain circulation is seen in many different diseases and syndromes, especially in young adults. It can be the predominant manifestation of the disorder or one aspect of a more widespread connective tissue disease. Inflammatory vasculitis is common in polyarteritis nodosa, while in patients with systemic lupus erythematosus (SLE) it is exceedingly rare. The main source of stroke in patients with SLE is embolic, rather than local thrombotic, including emboli from Libman–Sacks endocarditis. Takayasu arteritis is a form of segmental giant-cell arteritis that causes stenosis and aneurysmal dilatation of large arteries, especially the aorta or its major branches, which can cause occlusion of the common or internal carotid arteries, with resultant cerebral infarction. In the elderly, branches of the external carotid arteries are more commonly affected than in younger patients ('temporal arteritis'). There are a number of other disorders that have a vasculitic component. Systemic vasculitis and secondary vasculitis associated with infection, drugs and lympho-proliferative disorders can involve the central nervous system (CNS). The very rare primary angiitis of the CNS (sometimes referred to as primary granulomatous angiitis) has a poor prognosis.

In young adults cervical artery dissection is considered the second most frequent cause of stroke. It is associated with around 10–20% of acute cerebrovascular events. The main predisposing factors are trauma and primary hereditary disease of the arterial wall (e.g. fibromuscular dysplasia, Ehlers–Danlos syndrome type IV, etc.). There are two main hypotheses for the pathomechanism of arterial dissection:

- A rupture of the intimal layer of the arterial wall with penetration of intraluminal blood into the wall
- A rupture within the connective tissue of the intramedial layer (including vasa vasorum) resulting in dissection of the wall.

Ischaemic stroke can be caused by occlusion of the true arterial lumen by the expanded vessel wall or by embolism from a thrombus within the true lumen. Dissections can occur in many arteries, including the internal carotid and the vertebral arteries. MRI techniques are replacing conventional angiography as the gold standard for diagnosing both extra and intracranial cerebral artery dissections. This is because MRI can show the intraluminal haematoma itself (see Figure 4.8).

4.6 Spinal cord ischaemia

Spinovascular disease is rare compared with cerebrovascular disease. It includes spinal cord infarction, haemorrhage, transient ischaemic attack, and venous disease. The clinical symptoms of spinovascular disease usually begin abruptly and vary in severity depending on the vessel affected and level of the lesion. The diagnosis is suspected by the patient's history with acute onset of sudden and severe, sometimes radiating back pain associated with bilateral weakness, paresthesias, and sensory loss, loss of sphincter control with hesitancy and inability to void or defecate. The diagnosis is made by MRI including DWI but can sometimes be difficult during the first days because DWI of artifacts and because conventional T1-/T2-weighted MRI is mostly unremarkable in the acute phase. Myelography, cerebrospinal fluid (CSF) analysis and spinal angiography are sometimes useful for differential diagnosis.

An ischaemic lesion of the spinal cord (Figure 4.9) usually involves the territory of the anterior spinal artery (the ventral two-thirds of the spinal cord). The common causes of spinal cord infarcts are

Fig 4.8 Carotid artery dissection.

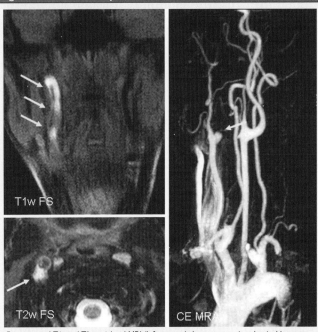

T1w FS

T2w FS

CE MR

Fat-saturated T1- and T2- weighted MRI (left; arrows) demonstrates intraluminal haematoma of the right ICA. Contrast enhanced MR angiography shows a proximal occlusion of the artery (right, arrow).

Fig 4.9 Spinal cord infarct.

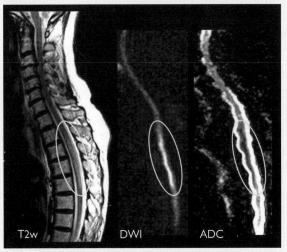

T2w

DWI

ADC

MRI demonstrates a large ischaemic lesion in the upper thoracic spinal cord (circle).

aortic disease (e.g. dissecting aneurysm, severe atherosclerosis, thrombosis) or surgical procedures such as aortic aneurysm repair, femoral artery catheterization, and coronary bypass grafting, small vessel disease related to inflammatory vasculopathy (e.g. polyarteritis nodosa, systemic lupus erythematodes, isolated CNS angiits), spinal or segmental artery compression or occlusion caused by disc fragments, extradural tumour or abscess, or sickle cell disease, hypotension caused by myocardial infarction or cardiac arrest; and spinal cord AVM.

References

Albers GW, Caplan LR, Easton JD, et al. (2002) TIA Working Group. Transient ischaemic attack—proposal for a new definition. *N Engl J Med* **347**, 1713–16.

Caplan LR, Hennerici M. (1998) Impaired clearance of emboli (washout) is an important link between hypoperfusion, embolism, and ischaemic stroke. *Arch Neurol* **55,** 1475–82.

Hennerici MG. (2004) The unstable plaque. *Cerebrovasc Dis* **17**(Suppl. 3), 17–22.

Johnston SC, Rothwell PM, Nguyen-Huynh MN, et al. (2007) Validation and refinement of scores to predict very early stroke risk after transient ischaemic attack. *Lancet* **369**, 283–92.

Mas JL, Arquizan C, Lamy C, et al. (2001) Recurrent cerebrovascular events associated with patent foramen ovale, atrial septal aneurysm, or both. *N Engl J Med* **345**, 1740–6.

Mohr JP. (1988) Cryptogenic stroke. *N Engl J Med* **318**, 1197–8.

Rolfs A, Martus P, Heuschmann PU, et al. (2011) Protocol and Methodology of the Stroke in Young Fabry Patients (sifap1) Study: A Prospective Multicenter European Study of 5,024 Young Stroke Patients Aged 18-55 Years. *Cerebrovasc Dis* **31**, 253–62.

Schievink W. (2001) Spontaneous dissection of the carotid and vertebral arteries. *N Engl J Med* **344**, 898–906.

The LADIS Study Group. (2011) 2001–2011: A decade of the LADIS (Leukoarasiosis And DISability) study: What have we learned about white matter changes and small-vessel disease?. *Cerebrovasc Dis* **32**, 577–588.

Chapter 5

Phenomenology of intracerebral haemorrhage

> **Key points**
>
> - Spontaneous ICH accounts for 10–15% of all strokes and is associated with a higher mortality rate than ischaemic stroke. Common causes include hypertension, cerebral amyloid angiopathy, coagulopathy, vascular anomalies, tumours, and various drugs.
> - The most important cause of spontaneous ICH is hypertension being the single greatest modifiable risk factor. The relative risk for ICH in hypertensive individuals is 3.9–13.3 times that of normotensive individuals. The risk is particularly high with non-compliance to antihypertensive treatment.
> - Spontaneous ICH is characterized by vessel rupture leading to extravasation of blood into the brain parenchyma. The size of the haematoma markedly increases in up to 40% of patients in the initial phase.

5.1 Classification and pathophysiology

Spontaneous intracerebral haemorrhage (ICH) is a blood clot that arises in the brain parenchyma in the absence of trauma or surgery. ICH accounts for 10–15% of all strokes and is associated with a higher mortality rate than either ischaemic stroke or subarachnoid haemorrhage. Common causes include hypertension, cerebral amyloid angiopathy (CAA), coagulopathy, vascular anomalies, tumours, and various drugs. Hypertension is the single greatest modifiable risk factor for ICH.

ICH can be classified into primary or secondary ICH according to the aetiology (Table 5.1). Primary ICH accounts for approximately 70-80% of cases and is characterized by the absence of an obvious underlying condition. It is caused by microvascular changes, especially in hypertension and alterations of the ageing brain (i.e. CAA). Secondary ICH is associated with anticoagulation or coagulopathy,

Table 5.1 Aetiology of spontaneous intracerebral haemorrhage		
Primary ICH	Hypertension	
	Cerebral amyloid angiopathy	
Secondary ICH	Aneurysm	Saccular Fusiform Mycotic
	Vascular malformation	AVM Cavernous malformation Venous angioma Dural arteriovenous fistula
	Neoplasm	Primary Metastatic
	Coagulopathy	Acquired Congenital
	Drugs	Alcohol Cocaine, amphetamine, ecstasy Sympathomimetics
	Haemorrhagic transformation of ischaemic stroke	
	Cerebral venous thrombosis	
	Vasculitis/vasculopathy	
	Pregnancy	Eclampsia Cerebral venous thrombosis
	Other / unknown	

alcohol, drug abuse, vasculitis and structural lesions (neoplasm, aneurysm, vascular malformations, etc).

Spontaneous ICH is characterized by vessel rupture leading to extravasation of blood into the brain parenchyma. The initial haematoma causes an increase in local pressure and subsequent rupture of other vessels surrounding the haematoma. Serial examinations have shown that in the initial phase, particularly during the first hours, the size of the haematoma markedly increases in up to 40% of patients. The presence of coagulation disorders and elevated blood pressure are predisposing factors for early haematoma growth and rebleeding. ICH growth is stopped by increasing counter pressure from the surrounding tissue and by haemostasis or, in large haematomas, from the elevated intracranial pressure.

After ICH occurs, mediators from the blood can induce an inflammatory reaction in and around the haematoma. Neutrophils, macrophages, leukocytes, and activated microglia can be found. The release of cytotoxic enzymes, free oxygen radicals, nitric oxide, and products of the phospholipid cascade is thought to contribute to secondary neural injury and cell death. Both necrotic and apoptotic neuronal death appear to play a role. The expression of matrix metalloproteinase 9, a proteolytic enzyme involved in re-organization of the extracellular matrix, has been shown to be increased following ICH.

In the tissue surrounding the haematoma, mechanical compression and release of mediators from the haematoma cause a marginal zone of ischaemia and oedema. These mechanisms are related to the frequent clinical deterioration early after ICH. There is controversy whether secondary ischaemia contributes to brain injury after ICH.

5.2 Primary ICH

5.2.1 Hypertensive intracerebral haemorrhage

The most important cause of primary ICH is hypertension, which continues to be the single greatest modifiable risk factor for ICH. The relative risk of ICH in hypertensive individuals is 3.9–13.3 times that of normotensive individuals. The risk of ICH is particularly high with non-compliance to antihypertensive treatment.

The most frequent sites of hypertensive ICH are the basal ganglia, thalamus, subcortical white matter of the cerebral lobes, cerebellum, and brainstem (Figure 5.1). This topographical distribution is due to the preferential histopathological changes in small penetrating arteries and arterioles arising directly from the main arterial trunks in the deep white matter and the retina that can be found in chronic hypertension. Due to hyalinization, fibrinoid change and subintimal fat deposition, small vessels show luminal occlusion or structural weakening, sometimes with dilatation and micro-aneurysms. Furthermore, reduced luminal energy supply in small vessels due to altered permeability of the arterial wall may lead to vessel ischaemia. These histopathological changes could cause rupture of the small vessels.

5.2.2 Cerebral amyloid angiopathy

CAA, another cause of primary ICH, accounts for 10% of cases. CAA represents an important cause of lobar ICH in elderly populations.

Fig 5.1 Hypertensive ICH.

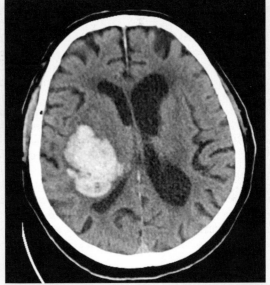

CT of a hypertensive ICH—typical lateral putaminal site of origin with a mass effect displacing the capsule medially and bearing on the thalamus.

CAA-related haemorrhages often recur within months or years, and associated imaging findings such as cerebral microbleeds and white matter disease can often be demonstrated (Figure 5.2). The microvascular changes are attributed to the pathological deposition of beta-amyloid in the media and adventitia of small cortical and leptomeningeal arteries and arterioles, explaining the preferential occurrence of lobar haemorrhage. Amyloid protein is a by-product of aberrant protein synthesis. These changes may be found in hereditary CAA of various forms, in healthy elderly people and in patients with neurodegenerative diseases (e.g. Alzheimer's disease, diffuse Lewy body disease, and vascular dementia). Fibrinoid degeneration, replacement of contractile elements and micro-aneurysms, which all lead to increased fragility of the vessels, have been proposed as possible pathomechanisms.

5.3 **Secondary ICH**

5.3.1 **Vascular anomalies**

Vascular anomalies are the second most common cause of ICH overall. Aneurysms, AVMs, cavernomas, dural arteriovenous fistulas,

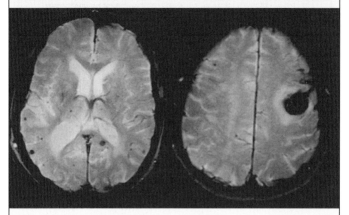

Fig 5.2 Cerebral amyloid angiopathy.

T2* weighted MRI of a patient with suspected CAA demonstrating lobar haemorrhage and multiple cerebral microbleeds.

and venous malformations all can result in secondary ICH. Most malformations occur in the hemispheres, although brainstem, cerebellar, or intraventricular lesions also exist. Most arteriovenous and cavernous malformations are single and sporadic, but they can also be multiple via an autosomal dominant inheritance. The annual risk of ICH is 1–4% for arteriovenous malformations, whereas cavernous and venous malformations have a minor risk of bleeding (approximately 0.2%). Cerebral venous malformations are assumed to be congenital lesions resulting from aberrant venous maturation. These entities have also been termed venous angiomas or developmental venous anomalies. Although rarely associated with ICH, venous malformations are the most frequently occurring vascular lesion demonstrated in autopsy and radiological series.

5.3.2 **Anticoagulation and coagulopathies**

Congenital (e.g. haemophilia) or acquired (e.g. in liver cirrhosis) coagulopathies of different aetiologies also cause ICH. The risk of ICH is increased 5–10-fold in patients anticoagulated with heparin or warfarin, even if the dosage is adjusted according to the international normalized ratio (INR). Advanced age, previous ischaemic stroke, hypertension, and intensity of anticoagulation further increase the risk of ICH. ICH occurs significantly more often in anticoagulated patients with leukoaraiosis or CAA. The risk of ICH in patients taking aspirin is much lower than estimated at 0.1%–0.2% (Antiplatelet Trialists' Collaboration 1994, Sandercock et al. 2003). The risk may be additionally increased in patients with very low cholesterol levels

55

or hypertension. In a meta-analysis of aspirin trials involving 55,462 participants, aspirin was associated with a slight absolute risk increase of haemorrhagic stroke. This was outweighed, however, by the overall risk reduction in myocardial infarction and ischaemic stroke. Use of other non-steroidal anti-inflammatory drugs does not seem to be associated with an overall increased risk of ICH.

After systemic fibrinolytic therapy for acute myocardial infarction, acute pulmonary embolism, deep vein thrombosis, or arterial and graft occlusion, the frequency of ICH is increased, but seldom higher than 2%. However, after systemic and intra-arterial fibrinolysis for cerebral infarction the risk of parenchymatous haemorrhage is markedly increased (7–9% after i.v. thrombolysis in SITS-MOST). Moreover, the risk of haemorrhagic transformation or symptomatic parenchymatous haemorrhage within an ischaemic infarct is increased in patients receiving heparin of any type.

5.3.3 **Haemorrhagic cerebral ischaemia**

Haemorrhagic cerebral ischaemia is a frequent finding in patients with territorial infarction, particularly after thrombolytic treatment or under anticoagulation. CT-based graduations can be used to describe the severity of haemorrhagic cerebral ischaemia: haemorrhagic transformation with only small or slightly confluent petechiae within the zone of ischaemic infarction; this was termed haemorrhagic infarction (HI), whereas parenchymal haemorrhage (PH) is defined by a space occupying effect. Among 800 acute stroke patients in ECASS II, haemorrhagic transformation (combined HI and PH) was found in 29.5% of alteplase treated patients within the first 4 days after symptom onset vs. 18.5% in the placebo group using these CT-based criteria. Mild HI frequently remains asymptomatic and is associated with relatively small infarcts, which have a good prognosis. More dense and extended haemorrhagic transformation and immediate PH is associated with delayed reperfusion and often large space-occupying infarcts, indicating a poor prognosis.

Although the pathomechanism of HI remains speculative, a disruption of the blood–brain barrier and leakage from ischaemic vascular endothelium have been proposed to precede haemorrhagic transformation. Dose-dependent side effects of alteplase treatment have been discussed as a risk factor. Animal models show damage of the microvascular basal lamina in alteplase treated rats, possibly due to increased co-activation of matrix metalloproteinases. Early blood–brain barrier disruption and reperfusion— either spontaneous when the previously occluded vessel recanalized, or after thrombolysis, causing extravasation in ischaemic tissue due to microvascular damage—are associated with HT after stroke.

5.3.4 **Alcohol and drugs**

In addition to its damaging effects on many organs, severe alcohol consumption is also an independent risk factor for ICH. Alcohol is thought to cause ICH by increasing the blood pressure and by affecting the coagulation system with disturbances of clotting factors in liver dysfunction and thrombocytopenia. Drugs such as cocaine, amphetamines and sympathomimetics have been associated with ICH by their secondary effects, which include hypertension, vasoconstriction, vasculitis, and infective endocarditis.

5.3.5 **Neoplasms**

ICH due to intracerebral neoplasms is relatively uncommon (0.5–5.8% of all ICH) and is probably due to tumour-related effects on the cerebral arteries or rupture of immature vessels. Haemorrhage is more likely with certain types of tumours, including glioblastoma, hemangioblastoma, oligodendroglioma, and metastatic tumours. Metastatic tumours at risk for secondary haemorrhage are malignant melanoma, renal cell, prostate, and lung cancer.

References

Antiplatelet Triallists' Collaboration. (1994) Collaborative overview of randomised trials: Prevention of death, myocardial infarction, and stroke by prolonged antiplatelet therapy in various categories of patients. *BMJ* **308**, 81–106.

Brott T, Broderick J, Kothari R, et al. (1997) Early haemorrhage growth in patients with intracerebral haemorrhage. *Stroke* **28**, 1–5.

Hart RG, Boop BS, Anderson DC. (1995) Oral anticoagulants and intracranial haemorrhage. Facts and hypotheses. *Stroke* **26**, 1471–7.

Knudsen KA, Rosand J, Karluk D, Greenberg SM. (2001) Clinical diagnosis of cerebral amyloid angiopathy: validation of the Boston criteria. *Neurology* **56**, 537–9.

Little JR, Dial B, Belanger G, Carpenter S. (1979) Brain haemorrhage from intracranial tumor. *Stroke* **10**, 283–8.

Lovelock CE, Cordonnier C, Naka H, et al. (2010) Antithrombotic drug use, cerebral microbleeds, and intracerebral hemorrhage: a systematic review of published and unpublished studies. *Stroke* 41, 1222–8.

Molina CA, Alvarez-Sabin J, Montaner J, et al. (2002) Thrombolysis-related haemorrhagic infarction: a marker of early reperfusion, reduced infarct size, and improved outcome in patients with proximal middle cerebral artery occlusion. *Stroke* **33**, 1551–6.

Rigamonti D, Hadley MN, Drayer BP, et al. (1988) Cerebral cavernous malformations. Incidence and familial occurrence. *N Engl J Med* **319**, 343–7.

Sandercock PA, Counsell C, Gubitz GJ, Tsong MC. Antiplatelet therapy for acute ischaemic stroke. *Chocrane Database Syst Rev.* 2008 Jul 16; (3) CD000029.

Sloan MA, Kittner SJ, Rigamonti D, Price TR. (1991) Occurrence of stroke associated with use/abuse of drugs. *Neurology* **41**, 1358–64.

Wahlgren N, Ahmed N, Davalos A, et al. (2007) Thrombolysis with alteplase for acute ischaemic stroke in the Safe Implementation of Thrombolysis in Stroke-Monitoring Study (SITS-MOST): an observational study. *Lancet* **369**, 275–82.

Yamada M. (2000) Cerebral amyloid angiopathy: an overview. *Neuropathology* **20**, 8–22.

Chapter 6

Phenomenology of subarachnoid haemorrhage and cerebral venous thrombosis

6.1 Subarachnoid haemorrhage

The incidence of subarachnoid haemorrhage (SAH) is 10.5 per 100,000 people per year. SAH is the cause of stroke in approximately 10% of patients. The aetiology of SAH can be classified into aneurysmal and non-aneurysmal. Intracranial aneurysms are the cause of 80% of SAH, followed by cerebral or spinal angioma, and other arteriovenous malformations (10%). The aetiology of the remaining 10% is diverse, and includes trauma and rare causes, such as arteriopathy (arterial dissection, cerebral amyloid angiopathy, kongophilic angiopathy, eclampsia, lupus, hypertension), blood or coagulation disorders, infection (bacterial meningitis, viral encephalitis, particularly herpes simplex), intoxication (alcohol, amphetamines, ecstasy, cocaine, sympathomimetic drugs), altitude sickness, or strangulation.

6.1.1 **Aneurysmal SAH**

The main cause of SAH is rupture of saccular aneurysms (Figure 6.1). In the older literature, saccular aneurysms are sometimes called 'congenital', which is misleading because the aneurysm develops during the course of life, enlarging over years to decades to become symptomatic in young and middle-aged patients. Why some patients develop aneurysms and others do not is largely unknown. It is supposed that unknown hereditary defects in the tunica media of the vessel wall determine the appearance of saccular aneurysms; this has been suggested because of a higher association of multiple aneurysms in Scandinavian populations. Saccular aneurysms are the most frequent type of aneurysm. They are typically located at the bifurcations of the major cerebral arteries of the circle of Willis (Figure 6.2). Histological examinations reveal a defect in the muscularis layer of the media lamina at the bifurcations of the arteries. If there is additional damage of the internal elastic lamina, the aneurysm forms

Fig 6.1 Subarachnoid haemorrhage.

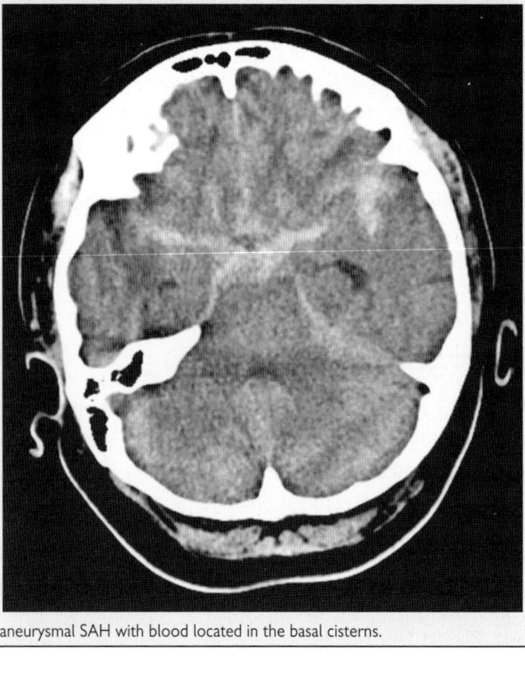

CT of aneurysmal SAH with blood located in the basal cisterns.

Fig 6.2 Typical sites of cerebral aneurysms.

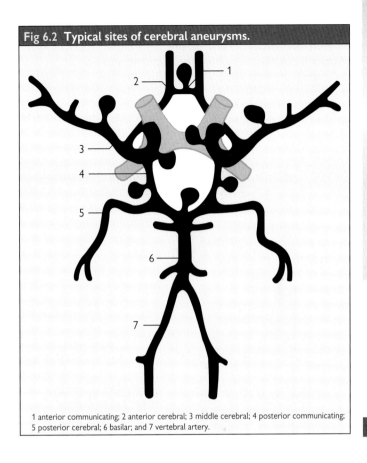

1 anterior communicating; 2 anterior cerebral; 3 middle cerebral; 4 posterior communicating;
5 posterior cerebral; 6 basilar; and 7 vertebral artery.

through this defect and may enlarge over time due to the high arterial flow and pressure. There is no definitive evidence that genetic factors and developmental abnormalities are the only cause for the development of saccular aneurysms. Saccular aneurysms are almost never found in neonates and are rare in children. It is likely that acquired risk factors such as arterial hypertension, smoking or alcohol abuse contribute to the formation of the aneurysm. Genetically determined disorders associated with aneurysms include Marfan's syndrome, Ehlers–Danlos disease, Neurofibromatosis type 1 and autosomal dominant polycystic kidney disease.

6.1.2 **Unruptured intracranial aneurysms**

Asymptomatic aneurysms may be present in 1% of the general adult population. To date, it is not possible to predict the course of an asymptomatic, incidental aneurysm with certainty. The average yearly risk of rupture is 1–2%, with an increased incidence for aneurysms with an internal diameter of 10 mm or greater. According to the International Study of Unruptured Intracranial Aneurysms (ISUIA), the risk of recurrent SAH in patients with a history of SAH is 0.5–2.4% per year (Figure 6.3). Besides the low risk of rupture with subsequent SAH, they may lead to neurological deficits due to compression of the brainstem or cranial nerves in the cavernous sinus (cranial nerves II, III, IV, VI).

Fig 6.3 Probability of SAH over time in patients with intracranial aneurysms (adapted from Wiebers et al, 2003).

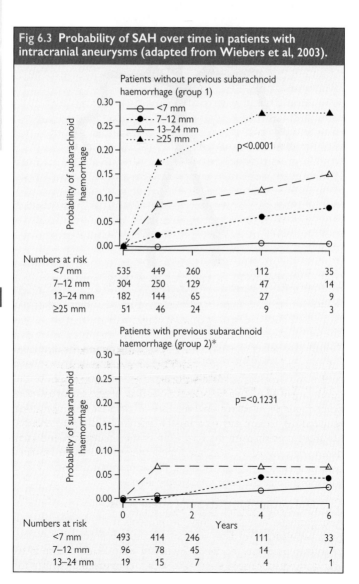

Fusiform aneurysms are a complication of advanced arteriosclerosis. They occur most frequently in the intracranial part of the internal carotid artery or in the basilar artery. Dolicho-ectatic intracranial arteries may cause a variety of neurological complications, including cerebral ischemia, cranial nerve and brain tissue compression, and hydrocephalus. Mechanisms involved in cerebral ischemia due to dolicho-ectatic intracranial arteries are: thrombotic occlusion of penetrating vessels, embolism to downstream vascular territories and obstruction of large vessels. The incidence of dolicho-ectatic intracranial arteries is estimated at approximately 1%. The vertebrobasilar system is most frequently involved.

6.1.3 **Non-aneurysmal SAH**

Non-aneurysmal perimesencephalic SAH represent approximately 10% of cases. It is characterized by mild symptoms at onset, subarachnoidal blood in the cisterns around the midbrain, and absence of aneurysms. The clinical course of perimesencephalic haemorrhage is uneventful and the outcome is good. The source of the haemorrhage is unclear; several studies propose venous or capillary leak (e.g. basal vein of Rosenthal, anterior longitudinal pontine, or interpeduncular and posterior communicating veins), lenticulostriate or thalamoperforating arteries, or cryptic brain stem arteriovenous malformations. In the absence of aneurysms, as evidenced from four-vessel panarteriography, perimesencephalic bleeding may be considered.

6.2 **Cerebral venous thrombosis**

For many years, thrombosis of the cerebral veins or venous sinus was considered a very rare disease with an invariably lethal course. This was because the diagnosis could be established only by post mortem examination. Today, modern neuroimaging including CT and MRI venography are widely available and establish the diagnosis in many patients with a benign course. As a rough estimate, 0.5–1% of stroke patients have a CVT. The aetiology of CVT is diverse, and many conditions have been associated with CVT. The most common manifestations are lateral, superior sagittal, inferior or superior petrosal, and cavernous sinus thrombosis. CVT may be bland (Figure 6.4) or may cause oedema and haemorrhagic infarction due to venous congestion. Isolated cortical vein thrombosis may mimic subarachnoid haemorrhage and is very difficult to diagnose *in vivo*. CT and MR venography may be normal due to rapid compensation of the filling defect by venous collaterals and recanalization (Figure 6.5).

6.2.1 **Idiopathic CVT**

In patients with non-septic CVT, nearly all conditions associated with a hypercoagulable state have been identified as risk factors.

Fig 6.4 Cerebral venous thrombosis.

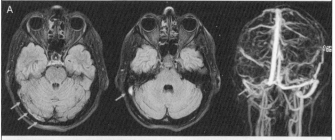

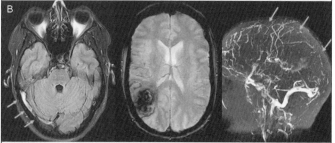

Cerebral venous thrombosis may either bland or with haemorrhagic infarction.
(A) Thrombosis of the right transverse sinus without structural abnormalities of the brain parenchyma. (B) Thrombosis of the superior sagittal sinus and right transverse sinus with subsequent haemorrhage in the right occipital and parietal lobe.

Fig 6.5 Isolated cortical venous thrombosis mimicking SAH.

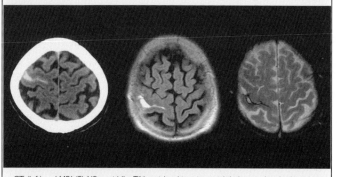

CT (left) and MRI (FLAIR—middle; T2* weighted imaging—right) show isolated subarachnoid haemorrhage in the right central sulcus. Cortical venous thrombosis was confirmed by digital subtraction angiography.

The most frequent hypercoagulation syndromes are activated protein C-resistance in factor V Leiden mutation and prothrombin-G20210A-mutations. These conditions should be meticulously searched for all in patients with idiopathic CVT because their presence may be relevant for acute treatment and long-term prevention of venous thrombosis for the patient and their family, if hereditary. CVT is a rare, but characteristic complication of pregnancy. In most affected patients it occurs during the post-partum period and is less common during the third trimester. CVT should therefore be considered in every woman presenting with new CNS symptoms around childbirth. Oral contraceptives have been extensively discussed as risk factors for CVT and other forms of thrombosis. In general, the risk of CVT from oral contraceptives is very small. However, the risk may considerably increase if other risk factors are present. Therefore, other risk factors (smoking, coagulation abnormalities, etc.) have to be systematically looked for. Even after a careful diagnostic evaluation, the proportion of patients with unknown aetiology remains relatively high (approximately 25%). Unlike with deep venous thrombosis (DVT), obesity is not a risk factor for CVT.

6.2.2 **Infectious CVT**
Infectious CVT most frequently originates from purulent local infections. Due to their close proximity, otitis media or mastoid infections predispose to thrombosis of the transverse and sigmoid sinus. Patients with infections of the ethmoidal or sphenoidal sinuses, other infections in the middle third of the face or dental abscesses may develop septic sinus cavernosus thrombosis. Most thromboses due to acute purulent infections are caused by *Staphylococcus aureus*, whereas in chronic infections, Gram-negative rods or fungi, such as *Aspergillus* spp. are more common. Metastatic septic CVT in patients with systemic infections, such as infectious endocarditis, is rare.

References

Bousser MG. (2000) Cerebral venous thrombosis: diagnosis and management. *J Neurol* **247**, 252–8.

Forget TR, Jr., Benitez R, Veznedaroglu E, et al. (2001) A review of size and location of ruptured intracranial aneurysms. *Neurosurgery* **49**, 1322–5.

Schwartz TH, Solomon RA. (1996) Perimesencephalic nonaneurysmal subarachnoid haemorrhage: review of the literature. *Neurosurgery* **39**, 433–40.

Urban P, Muller-Forell W. (2005) Clinical and neuroradiological spectrum of isolated cortical vein thrombosis. *J Neurol* **252**, 1476–81.

Wiebers DO, Whisnant JP, Huston J, 3rd, et al. (2003) Unruptured intracranial aneurysms: natural history, clinical outcome, and risks of surgical and endovascular treatment. *Lancet* **362**, 103–10.

Diagnosis and diagnostic instruments

Chapter 7

Clinical diagnosis

> **Key points**
> - In stroke patients certain combinations of neurologic signs may establish the location of ischemia and the vascular territory involved. Knowledge of the major arterial syndromes may also be helpful in identifying possible underlying stroke mechanisms.
> - The spectrum of clinical signs of intracerebral haemorrhage is very wide and reflects the location and size of the haematoma. Clinically, intracerebral haemorrhage cannot be distinguished from cerebral ischaemia.
> - The clinical syndrome of subarachnoid haemorrhage consists of severe headache of sudden onset ('thunderclap'), followed by loss of consciousness, nuchal rigidity, and few neurological deficits.
> - Cerebral venous thrombosis may be bland or may cause haemorrhagic infarction due to venous congestion. Depending on the location of the thrombosis and the collateral blood flow, the range of clinical symptoms is extremely wide.

7.1 Arterial stroke syndromes: anterior circulation

With a careful history and examination, the neurologist can often localize the region of brain damage or dysfunction. Particularly helpful is the knowledge of syndromes typical for an arterial distribution. In this chapter, clinical aspects of each of the commonly involved arteries—the vascular syndromes—are described.

7.1.1 Internal carotid artery territory
Occlusive disease of the ICA can cause transient attacks of monocular blindness (amaurosis fugax) described as dimming or darkening from above due to decreased blood flow through the ophthalmic

artery or micro-embolism into small ipsilateral retinal arteries. Brief episodes of hemispheral ischaemia can occur in critical stenosis with low flow in patients with haemodynamic compromise due to poor collateralization. In addition, emboli distal blockage of branches of the ACA or MCA, with longer lasting attacks. Occlusion of the ICA may remain asymptomatic or produce a large infarction in the MCA and ACA territories. Depending on the size of the affected brain tissue a spectrum of clinical syndromes can occur (see below). The final clinical picture depends upon the patency of collaterals, the speed of occlusion and recanalization as well as the individual vascular anatomy.

7.1.2 **Middle cerebral artery territory**

Complete MCA infarction is a life-threatening event and causes drowsiness, deviation of the head and eyes away from the hemiplegic side, contralateral hemiplegia of face, arm, and leg, hemisensory loss, and homonymous hemianopia. Dominant hemisphere lesions produce various aphasias while non-dominant hemisphere lesions produce contralateral neglect with anosognosia, aprosody, dysarthria, constructional impairment and spatial disorientation.

Vascular occlusions of the upper division of the MCA that supplies the frontal and superior parietal lobes lead to contralateral hemiparesis with a brachiofacial predominance and relative sparing of the lower extremity, contralateral hemisensory loss in a matching distribution, conjugate eye deviation or gaze preference, and neglect of contralateral side of space. Broca's aphasia with non-fluent speech, impaired repetition ability and relatively spared comprehension accompanies dominant hemisphere lesions. Buccofacial apraxia and ipsilateral-limb ideomotor apraxia are also common. In upper trunk infarcts in the right hemisphere patients frequently exhibit hemispatial neglect and abnormalities in the production of emotional prosody.

Patients with occlusion of the inferior trunk of the MCA that usually supplies the lateral surface of the temporal lobe and inferior parietal lobule usually have no elementary motor or sensory abnormalities. They often have a visual field defect, either a contralateral homonymous hemianopia or, more often, an upper quadrant anopsia of the contralateral visual field. Dominant hemisphere involvement leads to Wernicke-type aphasia, with impaired comprehension and repetition, but fluent speech that makes little sense and frequent semantic paraphasic errors. When the non-dominant hemisphere is affected contralateral hemineglect with a sensory predominance, anosognosia, constructional impairment, and difficulty in comprehending emotional prosody occurs. If the dominant angular gyrus is affected, Gerstmann's syndrome with difficulty telling right from left and naming digits, dyspraxia, agraphia, and problems calculating may be present.

Very small cortical lesions in the hand motor area of the precentral gyrus (termed the 'handknob') due to embolic distal Rolandic artery obstruction can cause acute ischaemic distal arm paresis. Partial hand knob lesions seem to indicate a somatotopic distribution of the hand motor cortex, which is not evident in larger lesions involving both lateral and medial zones of the hand knob.

Occlusion of the main middle cerebral artery stem before its lenticulostriate branches causes deep infarction of the middle cerebral artery territory termed striatocapsular infarct damaging the basal ganglia, the lateral part of the internal and external capsules, and less commonly the capsula extrema. Rostrally, the infarct may extend into the corona radiata. The typical clinical syndrome of pure striatocapsular infarct is a severe motor (or sensorimotor) hemiparesis or hemiplegia with or without dysarthria. Depending on the size and site of the lesion, the paresis predominantly involves the face and arm or the entire contralateral side. The quality of the deficit is mostly motor, although occasionally it may also be sensory or mixed. Adequate collateral circulation over the convexities in some cases prevents additional cortical infarction (see Table 7.1).

Small infarctions (most commonly <15mm) limited to the territory of one of the single perforators (single lenticulostriate arteries) are called lacunar strokes. Clinicopathological correlations indicate several clearly defined "lacunar syndromes" (see Table 7.2).

7.1.3 **Anterior cerebral artery territory**

Infarcts of the ACA territory are less common than middle cerebral artery territory infarcts. Some ACA infarcts are due to occlusive disease of the internal carotid artery. At times, both ACAs are supplied by one ICA and, in some cases, distal ACA branches supply both hemispheres causing bilateral ischaemia.

One of the most typical findings in ACA territory infarcts are weakness of the foot and leg, and to a lesser degree, paresis of the arm, with the face and tongue largely spared. Slight sensory impairments may be present in the affected half of the body. Acute ischaemic distal leg paresis might be caused by small cortical lesions in the precentral gyrus due to embolic obstruction of the paracentral lobule artery. An ischaemic cause—as opposed to peripheral nerve palsy—should especially be taken into consideration in patients with acute onset of isolated distal leg paresis and lack of accompanying sensory deficits. If the supplementary motor cortex is affected, proximal paresis of the shoulder and hip muscles may occur and become apparent if alternating movements between right and left extremities are examined. If the left hemisphere is affected, a transcortical motor and sensory aphasia often results with muteness, reduced spontaneous output, but preserved repetition and normal articulation abilities. Urinary incontinence has been described as one of the

Table 7.1 Patterns of occlusion of the middle cerebral artery and their clinical manifestations

MCA lesion	Infarct on coronal image	Clinical manifestation
Entire territory	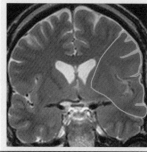	– Contralateral gaze palsy, hemiplegia, hemisensory loss, spatial neglect, hemianopia – Global aphasia (L) – May progress to malignant MCA stroke with coma
MCA stem	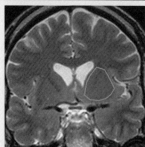	– Contralateral hemiplegia, hemisensory loss – Transcortical motor or sensory aphasia (L)
Superior division	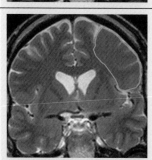	– Contralateral hemiplegia, hemisensory loss, gaze palsy – Broca's aphasia (L)
Inferior division	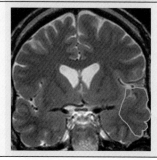	– Contralateral hemianopia or upper quadrant anopsia – Wernicke's aphasia (L) – Dyspraxia (R)

Table 7.2 Lacunar syndromes

	Symptoms	Location
Pure motor hemiparesis	Weakness of face, arm and leg	Internal capsule, pons
Pure sensory stroke	Sensory deficit of face, arm and leg	Thalamus
Motor-sensory stroke	Weakness and sensory deficit of face, arm, and leg	Internal capsule
Ataxic hemiparesis	Hemiparesis, ipsilateral ataxia	Internal capsule, pons
Dysarthria, clumsy hand	Dysarthria, clumsy hand	Internal capsule, pons

classic symptoms in unilateral or bilateral ACA occlusion. Patients with unilateral ACA or bilateral frontal infarcts commonly show akinetic mutism and abulia.

The recurrent artery of Heubner is one of the major branches of the ACA; it supplies the head of the caudate nucleus and the anterior limb of the internal capsule. Besides dysarthria, occlusion of this artery leads to behavioural changes: abulia, but also restlessness, hyperactivity, agitation, euphoria, and talkativeness have been reported.

7.2 **Arterial stroke syndromes: posterior circulation**

7.2.1 **Vertebral artery territory**

One of the most frequently reported symptoms in VA disease is dizziness, usually accompanied by brainstem signs, such as diplopia, oscillopsia, weakness, and numbness.

Occlusion of the intracranial VA or its main penetrating arteries that originate from the distal VA can produce the dorsolateral medullary syndrome (Wallenberg's syndrome). The lateral medullary area is also variably supplied by small branches arising from the posterior inferior cerebellar artery, the anterior inferior cerebellar artery, or the basilar artery. Important symptoms and signs of this syndrome are:

- Diziness, ataxia with vertigo and nystagmus
- Nausea and/or vomiting
- Loss of pin prick sensation on the ipsilateral side of the face and contralateral side of the body
- Horner's syndrome on the ipsilateral side
- Dysphagia and hoarseness due to paralysis of the ipsilateral vocal cord.

If patients have additional infarction in the ipsilateral inferior cerebellum (fed by the posterior inferior cerebellar artery) headache, head tilt, and in large lesions stupor can result. Involvement of the automatic respiratory centre may cause abnormal respiratory control.

Cerebellar lesions above the horizontal fissure are in the superior cerebellar artery territory, while those below are caused by disease of the anterior or posterior inferior cerebellar arteries. The syndrome of cerebellar infarction can be deceptively slight with vomiting, dizziness and gait ataxia. Space-occupying cerebellar lesions may compress the cerebellopontine angle causing lesions of the cranial nerves V, VI, VII, and VIII. Compression of the pons leads to conjugate gaze paresis to the ipsilateral side. This might lead to a life-threatening increase of posterior fossa pressure and to death from medullary compression. Small lesions in the cerebellum may cause little or no neurological deficits (see Table 7.3).

7.2.2 **Basilar artery territory**

The clinical features of occlusion of the BA depend on the rapidity of vessel occlusion, the location and extent of the thrombosis, and the adequacy of a collateral circulation. Basilar artery thrombosis may result in a devastating syndrome, with a very poor prognosis, involving tetraparesis, cranial nerve abnormalities, stupor, and coma. However, it may cause little or no deficit if anastomoses compensate for segmented occlusions, especially in the mid-portion. Transient and unstable, repeat ischaemic brainstem attacks with rapidly changing diplopia, dizziness, alternating weakness between limbs and headache are common signs prior to basilar artery thrombosis. The typical findings in patients with occlusion of the mid-basilar artery are: bilateral weakness (possibly alternating), bulbar or pseudobulbar palsy, abnormalities of eye movement, nystagmus, skew deviation, and coma. Small emboli to the distal basilar artery (top-of-the-basilar syndrome) cause pupillary and eye movement abnormalities, altered level of consciousness, and amnesia.

Occlusion of a single perforating branch of the basilar artery results in a restricted infarct in the brainstem, especially in the pons and in the mid-brain. Brainstem infarcts are distinguished by cranial nerve abnormalities on the ipsilateral side of the face, and paralysis or sensitive disturbances on the opposite side of the body (Weber's syndrome if the midbrain is involved and Millard–Gubler's syndrome if the pons is involved; see Table 7.4). Pure symptoms may occur, but overlaps and inconstant phenomenologies are quite frequent due to the highly variable vascular anatomy in different individuals.

7.2.3 **Posterior cerebral artery territory**

The most common finding in patients with PCA territory infarction is a visual field defect (contralateral homonymous hemianopia) due to affection of the striate cortex, the optic radiations, or to a deep

Table 7.3 Patterns of occlusion of the cerebellar arteries and their clinical manifestations

Cerebellar artery	Infarct on coronal image	Clinical manifestation
Posterior inferior cerebellar artery (from intracranial vertebral artery)	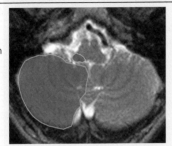	Dorsolateral medullary syndrome: Vertigo, nystagmus, Palsies of the V, IX, and X cranial nerves, ipsilateral Horner's syndrome, ataxia, contralateral loss of sensation for temperature and pain. When infarct spares the medulla: Vertigo, headache, gait ataxia, appendicular ataxia, horizontal nystagmus
Anterior inferior cerebellar artery (from lower basilar artery)	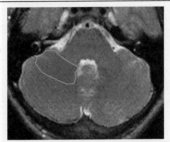	Vertigo, vomiting, tinnitus, dysarthria, dysphagia, ipsilateral conjugate-lateral gaze palsy. *Ipsilateral*: Limb motor weakness, facial palsy, hearing loss, trigeminal sensory loss, Horner's syndrome, dysmetria *Contralateral*: Loss of sensation for temperature and limb
Superior cerebellar artery (from upper basilar artery)	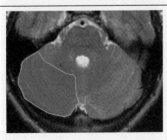	*Ipsilateral*: limb dysmetria, Horner's syndrome. *Contralateral*: loss of sensation for temperature and pain, IV nerve palsy, hearing loss

Table 7.4 Clinical signs in brainstem syndromes

III plus syndrome

Top of the basilar syndrome (common)	Infarct of mesencephalon, thalamus and occipital and temporal lobe: • Unconsciousness • Oculomotor disturbances • Cortical blindness • Neuropsychological and mnestic deficits.
Weber's syndrome (common)	Paramedian and lateral midbrain infarct: • Ipsilateral III nerve palsy • Contralateral hemiplegia.
Claude's syndrome (less common)	Infarct in the paramedian upper-midbrain and cerebro-thalamic connections: • Ipsilateral III nerve palsy • Contralateral cerebellar signs.
Benedikt's syndrome (less common)	Infarct in the paramedian upper-midbrain and red nucleus: • Ipsilateral III nerve palsy • Involuntary abnormal movements (tremor and chorea) affecting the contralateral limbs.

VI/VII plus syndrome

Foville's syndrome (common)	Infarct in the pontine tegmentum: • Ipsilateral horizontal-gaze palsy (supranuclear VI nerve palsy) • Contralateral hemiparesis.
Millard–Gubler's syndrome (rare)	Infarct in the base of the pons: • Ipsilateral VI nerve palsies • Ipsilateral complete VII palsies • Contralateral hemiplegia.

Lower brainstem syndrome

Wallenberg's syndrome (frequent)	Lateral medullary infarct (see Figure 8.3): • Ataxia • Vertigo • Nystagmus • Nausea and vomiting • Loss of pick sensation in the ipsilateral side of the face and contralateral side of the body • Difficulties in swallowing • Difficulties in phonation • Ipsilateral Horner's syndrome.

infarction involving the lateral geniculate body or the visual cortex. Positive symptoms, such as photopsias and visual illusion, particularly if the non-dominant hemisphere is affected, may also occur. Occlusion of the proximal (P1 segment) posterior cerebral artery can cause infarcts in the brainstem with accompanying hemiplegia or in the thalamus with hemisensory loss. Involvement of the hippocampus in posterior cerebral artery stroke may lead to deficits of long-term memory. Bilateral posterior cerebral artery territory infarction leads to cortical blindness, amnesia and agitation. These patients may not admit that they cannot see (Anton's syndrome).

Numerous vascular syndromes of the thalamus are known affecting the thalamic nuclei in different combinations with typical neurological syndromes (see Table 7.5). The main blood supply for the thalamus comes from the proximal segments of the posterior cerebral artery through the paramedian, the inferolateral, and the posterior choroidal arteries. The remaining parts receive their supply from the posterior communicating artery through the polar arteries. Four classical thalamic stroke territories are described: The most common thalamic infarcts involve either: the inferolateral (syn. thalamogeniculate) (1) or the paramedian (syn. thalamoperforant) (2) territories, the latter often

Table 7.5 Four main vascular territories of the thalamus and their clinical manifestations

Vascular territories of the thalamus	Clinical manifestation
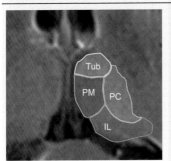	**Tuberothalamic infarcts (carotid territory)** Impairments of arousal and orientation, learning and memory, personality, and executive function; L: language deficits; R: visual-spatial deficits. **Paramedian infarcts (posterior circulation)** Decreased arousal, particularly if bilateral, impaired learning and memory: L: language deficits; R: visual-spatial deficits **Inferolateral infarcts (posterior circulation)** Contralateral hemisensory loss, hemiparesis and hemiataxia, and pain syndromes. **Posterior choroidal infarcts (posterior circulation)** Visual field deficits, sensory loss, weakness, and dystonia

77

involving the upper mid-brain, as well and may be bilateral. The third type is the posterior choroidal infarct (3), which has been reported rarely, compared to the third most common type of thalamic stroke, anterior (syn. Polar or tuberothalamic), (4) thalamic infarcts.

7.3 **Borderzone infarcts**

Borderzone infarctions located at the edges of vascular territories of the large cerebral arteries are a common infarction pattern in patients with occlusive artery disease or haemodynamic failure. The cerebral borderzones are divided into the superficial or cortical borderzones wedged between the territory of the ACA and the MCA, or between the MCA and the PCA territory and the deep or subcortical borderzone located in the vascular territory between superficial and deep arterial systems emerging of the MCA. A stuttering onset of clinical symptoms in borderzone infarcts over hours to days, sometimes worsening with hypotensive episodes, has been reported, whereas in other cases, an immediately complete or rapidly progressive presentation of clinical symptoms was seen. Altogether, patients with borderzone infarctions display the complete spectrum of symptoms of cerebral ischaemia. In anterior cortical borderzone infarcts crural hemiparesis, hemihypaesthesia, transcortical motor aphasia and less frequently word-finding difficulties can occur. Hemianopia, hemihypaesthesia, limb weakness, word-finding difficulty or transcortical aphasia, Wernicke-type aphasia and neuropsychological deficits like apraxia, agnosia, stupor, neglect, and poor short-term memory are often part of the clinical presentation in posterior cortical borderzone infarcts. In internal borderzone infarcts, motor and sensorimotor hemiparesis, language disturbance such as transcortical motor, sensory, mixed or unclassifiable aphasia and less frequently dysarthria and neuropsychological deficits like impaired verbal memory, higher-level naming, verbal abstract conceptual skills, visual memory as well as disturbed visuospatial, constructional and planning skills are found. Bilateral involvement is known to falsely mimic brainstem symptoms, e.g. the so-called man-in-the-barrel-syndrome with bi-brachial paralysis when affecting the anterior borderzones on both sides, and cortical blindness (Anton's syndrome) when affecting the posterior borderzones bilaterally (see Table 7.6).

7.4 **Intracerebral haemorrhage**

7.4.1 **Intracerebral haemorrhage**

The clinical signs of ICH range from mild to severe headache, different degrees of focal neurological deficits to disturbance of consciousness, and even coma. The pattern of clinical signs reflects the location and size of the ICH and indicate prognosis. Clinically, ICH cannot be distinguished from cerebral ischaemia, although a rapid onset, signs of increased intracerebral pressure and oedema (i.e. headache, vomiting, singultus, seizures and disturbance of consciousness) are more frequent.

The clinical presentation of putaminal haemorrhage may vary from relatively minor pure motor hemiparesis to severe weakness, sensory loss, eye deviation, hemianopia, aphasia and depressed level of consciousness due to disruption of connecting fibres in the subcortical white matter. These signs are clinically indistinguishable from ischaemia in these territories. Thalamic haemorrhage often presents with contralateral sensory loss. Due to the proximity of the internal capsule, motor defects are also common. Pupil and extra-ocular movement defects and impaired consciousness—due to effects on the rostral ascending activating system—may also be seen. Brainstem haemorrhage may present as coma, posturing, loss of brainstem reflexes, pupillary and oculomotor abnormalities, affection of other cranial nerves, cardiac arrhythmia, and respiratory insufficiency. It most commonly involves the pons and generally has a bad prognosis. Occasionally, symptomatic intracranial bleeding in the brainstem may derive from cavernoma and be limited in size. Cerebellar haemorrhage typically presents with abrupt onset of vertigo, headache, vomiting and inability to walk without presence of hemiparesis. This type of haemorrhage may act as a posterior fossa mass, producing hydrocephalus and/or brainstem compression. Therefore, in patients with cerebellar or large supratentorial haematoma, coma, pupillary abnormalities and respiratory insufficiency indicate secondary brainstem involvement and tentorial herniation.

The clinical spectrum of lobar haemorrhages depends on its location and size. Lobar ICH could lead to paresis (motor cortex), sensory deficits (sensory cortex), visual problems i.e. homonymous hemianopia (visual cortex), speech problems and mnestic and behavioural disturbances (temporal and frontal cortex). In some cases (particularly if the temporal lobes are affected) lobar haemorrhages may cause focal seizures, sometimes with secondary generalization.

7.4.2 **Cerebral amyloid angiopathy**

CAA is typically asymptomatic until spontaneous intracerebral haemorrhage occurs. Other features include dementia, seizures, cerebral ischaemia, transient ischaemic attacks, and leucoencephalopathy. CAA-related haemorrhages mostly occur in corticosubcortical (or lobar) brain regions and can extend through the cortex and the subarachnoid space or, less commonly, into the ventricles. CAA-related haemorrhages are typically multiple or recurrent, and this feature is important in the clinical diagnosis of the disorder. According to the Boston criteria, additional features for in vivo diagnosis of "probable CAA" include age over 55 years and no other cause of haemorrhage; histopathological analysis has validated these features. The definite diagnosis of CAA can only be made by post-mortem examination.

7.5 **Subarachnoid haemorrhage**

The clinical hallmark of an SAH is usually severe headache of sudden onset, typically developing within a split second, followed by loss of consciousness, nuchal rigidity and few neurological deficits.

Table 7.6 Borderzone infarction patterns and typical neurological symptoms			
Vascular lesion	**Infarction pattern**	**Clinical manifestation**
Cortical ACA/MCA	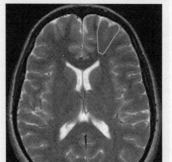	Crural hemiparesis, hemihypaesthesia Transcortical motor aphasia, word-finding difficulty
Cortical PCA/MCA	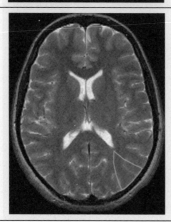	Hemianopia, hemihypaesthesia, limb weakness. Word-finding difficulty, transcortical aphasia, Wernicke-type aphasia. Neuropsychological deficits (apraxia, agnosia, stupor, neglect and poor short-term memory). Gerstmann's syndrome

(continued)

Table 7.6 (Cont'd) Borderzone infarction patterns and typical neurological symptoms

Subcortical MCA/ACA	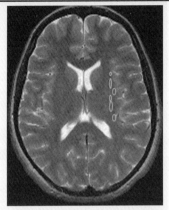	Motor and sensorimotor hemiparesis. Transcortical motor, sensory, mixed or unclassifiable aphasia. Dysarthria. Neuropsychological deficits (impaired verbal memory, higher-level naming, verbal abstract conceptual skills, visual memory, disturbed visuospatial, constructional, and planning skills)
Bilateral ACA/MCA cortical	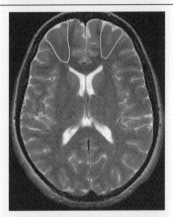	'Brainstem symptoms' (mimics) Man-in-the-barrel-syndrome
Bilateral PCA/MCA cortical	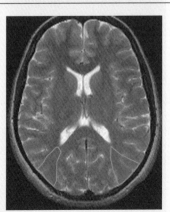	Anton's syndrome

Table 7.7 Hunt and Hess classification of SAH	
Grade	Description
0	Unruptured aneurysm
1	Asymptomatic ruptured aneurysm – Mild headache – Slight nuchal rigidity
2	No neurological deficit except for cranial nerve palsy – Moderate to severe headache – Nuchal rigidity
3	Drowsiness, confusion and/or focal neurological deficit
4	Stupor, moderate to severe neurological deficit
5	Deep coma, moribund appearance

Approximately half of patients with SAH lose consciousness initially. Most patients then regain consciousness spontaneously, so the clinical picture may resemble syncope of cardiac origin or suggest an epileptic seizure. However, seizures are also common at onset of or after SAH. The Hunt and Hess scale (Table 7.7) is still widely used to simplify and standardize the findings of the initial neurological examination. Focal neurological deficits may indicate the site of a ruptured aneurysm. A haematoma located in the Sylvian fissure indicates an MCA aneurysm, which leads to contralateral hemiparesis. This may be confirmed on CT, especially if this shows aneurysmatic bleeding. CT, however, is often unrevealing in subacute SAH. Lumbar puncture with CSF analysis is therefore mandatory if SAH is suspected clinically. Haematomas in the anterior interhemispheric cisterns are associated with ACA or anterior communicating artery aneurysms, causing mutism in some cases. Blood in the interpeduncular cisterns indicates a BA aneurysm. Clinically, this may mimic a basilar syndrome, or cause oculomotor palsy due to an aneurysm of the posterior communicating artery.

7.6 Cerebral venous thrombosis

Depending on the location of the thrombosis and the collateral blood flow, the range of clinical symptoms associated with CVT is extremely wide, and the clinical presentation is very variable and sometimes unspecific. With decreasing frequency, patients present with one of the following clinical syndromes: headache plus focal neurological deficits and focal seizures, isolated intracranial hypertension with headache and papillary oedema, sinus cavernosus syndrome with chemosis, protrusio bulbi and painful ophthalmoplegia, subacute unspecific encephalopathy, or isolated cranial nerve lesions with headache. Frequently, these syndromes overlap and none of the syndromes is specific for CVT.

The onset of symptoms is highly variable; approximately 50% of patients describe a subacute (two days to one month) occurrence of symptoms, while acute (two days or less) or chronic presentations (more than two months) are less frequent. Most patients describe their headache as dull and oppressive with a uni- or bilateral localization, often mimicking tension-type headache or migraine. Conversely, patients with CVT may occasionally present with an unusually severe headache of sudden onset; therefore CVT as well as SAH should be included in the differential diagnosis of patients with 'thunderclap headache'.

CVT associated seizures are typically difficult to treat; therefore, every patient with new therapy-resistant focal seizures or series of seizures including status epilepticus in combination with a focal deficit should be suspected of having a CVT. Because the clinical picture develops slowly and insidiously in most patients with CVT, the diagnosis is frequently overlooked during the initial clinical evaluation of patients complaining of headache and other non-specific neurological symptoms. It is not known how many cases of CVT remain undetected because the patient has minimal or no symptoms.

References

Bogousslavsky J, Caplan LR. (2001) *Stroke syndromes*, 2nd edn. Cambridge University Press, Cambridge.

Caplan LR. (1996) *Posterior Circulation Disease: Clinical Findings, Diagnosis, and Management.* Blackwell Science, Oxford.

Förster A, Szabo K, Hennerici MG. (2008) Pathophysiological concepts of stroke in hemodynamic risk zones—do hypoperfusion and embolism interact? *Nat Clin Pract Neurol.* **4**, 216–25.

Hennerici MG, Daffertshofer M, Caplan LR, Szabo K. (2007) *Case Studies in Stroke: Common and Uncommon Presentations.* Cambridge University Press, Cambridge.

Schmahmann JD. (2003) Vascular syndromes of the thalamus. *Stroke* **34**, 2264–78.

Plate 1 Global burden of stroke (source: WHO). See also Fig 1.1.

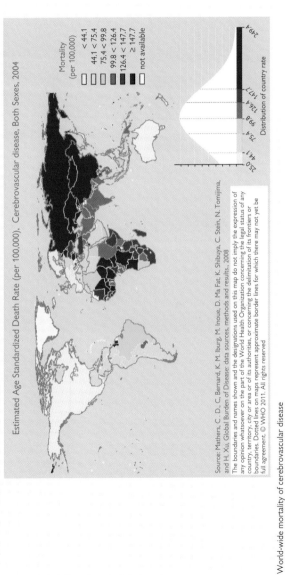

Estimated Age Standardized Death Rate (per 100,000), Cerebrovascular disease, Both Sexes, 2004

Mortality
(per 100,000)
□ < 44.1
□ 44.1 < 75.4
□ 75.4 < 99.8
■ 99.8 < 126.4
■ 126.4 < 147.7
■ ≥ 147.7
□ not available

Source: Mathers, C. D., C, Bernard, K. M. Iburg, M. Inoue, D. Ma Fat, K. Shibuya, C. Stein, N. Tomijima, and H. Xiu, Global Burden of Disease: data sources, methods and results, 2008

The boundaries and names shown and the designations used on this map do not imply the expression of any opinion whatsoever on the part of the World Health Organization concerning the legal status of any country, territory, city or area or of its authorities, or concerning the delimitation of its frontiers or boundaries. Dotted lines on maps represent approximate border lines for which there may not yet be full agreement.

World-wide mortality of cerebrovascular disease

Plate 2 Stroke in ICA stenosis. See also Fig 4.1.

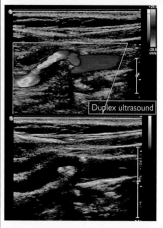
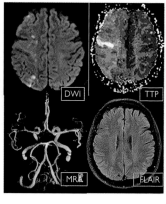

Proximal right ICA stenosis diagnosed by extracranial duplex ultrasound (left) with subsequent embolic infarction and extensive hypoperfusion (DWI and PWI, upper right) in the corresponding MCA territory.

Plate 3 Arterial spin labelling MRI techniques. See also Fig 8.8.

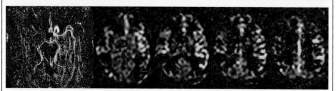

The colour-coded dynamic angiography map (left) describes the time point of maximum blood inflow to arterial vessels; warm colours (red and yellow) indicate early arrival of blood, whereas cold colours (green and blue) indicate later arrival. The figure shows an earlier arrival in the ipsilateral P1 segment and in the contralateral siphon in a patient with aright ICA occlusion. ASL perfusion maps show hypoperfusion in the right MCA territory.

Plate 4 Vascular imaging—ultrasound. See also Fig 8.9.

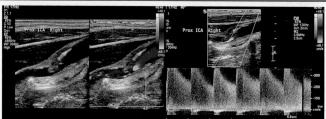

High-grade stenosis of the proximal right ICA as detected by B-mode and colour duplex ultrasound imaging.

Plate 5 Stroke—an emergency. See also Fig 10.2.

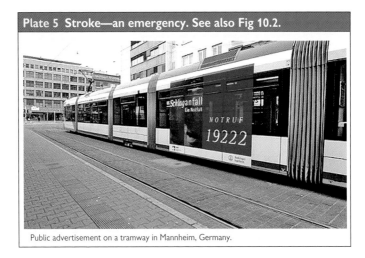

Public advertisement on a tramway in Mannheim, Germany.

Plate 6 Emergency CT in acute stroke. See also Fig 10.3.

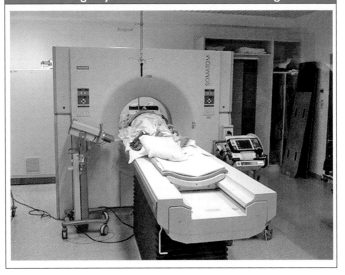

Chapter 8

Imaging in acute stroke

> **Key points**
> - CT scan of the brain performed in an emergency setting accurately identifies most cases of intracranial haemorrhage.
> - Diffusion-weighted MRI allows visualization of ischaemic lesions at very early time points and supplies information concerning lesion size, site, acuity as well as the possible aetiology.
> - A variety of modern MRI and ultrasound techniques can be used to further study tissue and vascular abnormalities in ischaemic stroke.
> - Several diagnostic tests should be performed routinely in patients with suspected ischaemic stroke to identify systemic conditions that may mimic or cause stroke or that may influence therapeutic options.

8.1 CT in acute stroke

8.1.1 Computed tomography

In most hospital settings a CT scan of the brain is the first line of imaging in order to differentiate between cerebral haemorrhage and infarction (and other conditions, such as tumours or abscesses). Parenchymal haemorrhage is easily seen as a hyperattenuated, space-occupying mass. Infarcts appear as lucencies relative to the density of the brain. However, in the acute phase of ischaemic stroke, particularly in the first 3h, but sometimes up to 48hr after onset of symptoms, abnormalities may be missed or be difficult to demonstrate on CT. Undeniable advantages of CT are a short acquisition time and the availability 24hr a day in smaller hospitals. Further disadvantages, however, are the radiation exposure and the low inter-rater reliability of diagnoses, particularly for acute ischaemic lesions and those located in the posterior circulation (brainstem and cerebellum). One of the first CT signs in hyperacute stroke is a subtle cortical hypodensity causing a loss of grey-white matter differentiation. There might also be

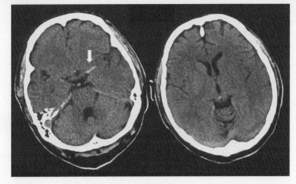

CT performed 4 hours after onset of a severe neurological deficit (NIHSS 18) shows signs of an acute infarction in the territory of the left MCA with a hyperdense MCA sign (white arrow), cortical effacement, edema in the lenticular nucleus and demarcation in the temporal lobe.

effacement of cortical sulci and obscuration of the lentiform nucleus. The hyperdence MCA sign is often associated with a proximal occlusion of the vessel and a large territorial MCA infarction in patients presenting with a severe neurological deficit. After 12-24 h, hypodensity of the infarcted area becomes visible and reaches its maximum at 3 to 5 days after onset (see Figure 8.1).

8.1.2 Computed tomographic angiography

CTA requires spiral CT techniques and the bolus injection of a contrast agent (see Figure 8.2). Even though it has not yet been well evaluated against the gold standard of selective intra-arterial catheter angiography, it does provide multiple viewing angles and three-dimensional reconstruction of the vascular tree, especially of the carotid arteries. However, the examination introduces the risk of allergic reaction and fluid overload in elderly patients with congestive heart failure.

8.2 **Magnetic resonance imaging**

Cerebral ischaemia is more easily and reliably detected with magnetic resonance imaging (MRI), particularly with diffusion-weighted MRI (DWI, see Figure 8.3). Therefore, in many stroke centres, MRI protocols are currently replacing CT as the initial radiological examination for the evaluation of patients with acute stroke. In all patients with acute stroke a routine MRI stroke protocol including T1-, T2-, FLAIR-, diffusion-, and perfusion-weighted images, as well as a time-of-flight magnetic resonance angiography (MRA) of the circle of Willis should

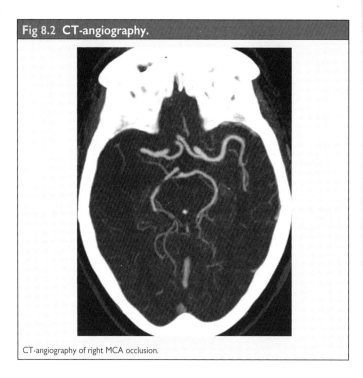

Fig 8.2 CT-angiography.

CT-angiography of right MCA occlusion.

be performed. If appropriately managed, this procedure does not cause a delay (15–20min).

8.2.1 Diffusion-weighted MRI

DWI is sensitive to changes of water molecule mobility and detects reduced proton mobility due to cytotoxic cell swelling, an early event in the cascade of ischaemic tissue change, before T2-weighted MRI shows abnormality. It provides a higher lesion-to-background contrast than conventional MRI, facilitating lesion detection in early stages of stroke, and allows differentiation of acute and chronic tissue change. The regional decrease of diffusion is visible as hyper-intensity on DWI images and as hypo-intensity on quantitative maps of the apparent diffusion coefficient (ADC). Current evidence suggests that restricted diffusion is caused by cell swelling associated with cytotoxic oedema formation with failure of energy dependent pumps and influx of sodium and calcium, possibly accentuated by metabolic stress due to peri-infarct depolarizations. A DWI study can typically be generated within 4–5sec. Using DWI early infarct pattern detection has dramatically simplified (see Figure 8.4).

8.2.2 Perfusion-weighted magnetic resonance imaging

Changes of cerebral blood flow and of cerebral microcirculation, the basic mechanisms underlying cerebral ischaemia, are not depicted

Fig 8.3 CT and MRI in a case of medullary stroke.

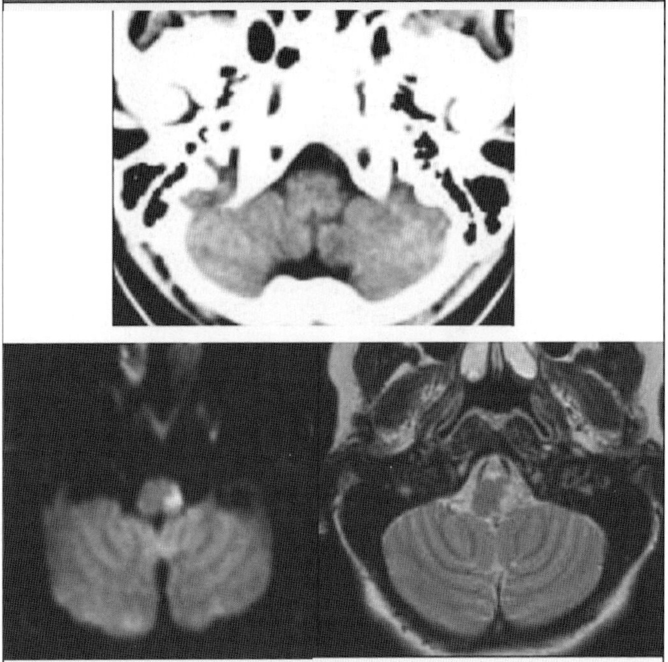

While computed tomography (CT) scan is unremarkable, DWI and T2 MRI show a hyperintense acute ischaemic lesion in the left dorsolateral medulla oblongata.

by DWI. Perfusion-weighted MRI (PWI) offers a means to obtain semiquantitative haemodynamic information in cerebral ischaemia with relatively high resolution and short acquisition times covering all cerebral vascular territories. In acute cerebral ischaemia, dynamic susceptibility contrast (DSC) MRI is the most widely evaluated technique. It uses information from transient local changes of magnetic field homogeneity (susceptibility effects) induced by the bolus passage of a paramagnetic contrast agent in dynamic T2*-weighted MRI acquisitions. The extent of haemodynamically compromised tissue is readily provided by the temporal characteristics of the contrast bolus arrival in 'time to peak' or 'mean transit time' maps (see Figure 8.5).

8.2.3 **Susceptibility-weighted T2* MRI**

Susceptibility-weighted MRI using T2*-sequences is increasingly applied in acute stroke protocols to detect haemorrhage. The high contrast of local signal loss caused by paramagnetic effects of deoxyhaemoglobin, even when present only in traces, facilitates lesion detection. The excellent accuracy of MRI including T2*-sequences in the detection of intracerebral haemorrhage—even very small microbleeds (see Figure 8.6)—has been confirmed in multiple studies. The phenomenon

Fig 8.4 Different patterns of infarction as detected by DWI.

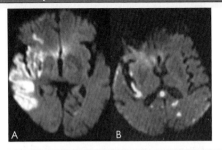
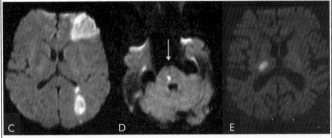

DWI detects typical infarct patterns: (A) Right territorial MCA stroke, (B) Multiple acute ischaemic lesions in different vascular territories suggesting a cardiac source of embolism, (C) Acute ischaemic lesions in the anterior and posterior borderzones suggesting stenosis of the ipsilateral ICA, (D) acute lacunar paramedian pontine stroke (arrow) and (E) acute ischaemic lacunar lesion of the right thalamus.

Fig 8.5 MRI characterization of acute stroke.

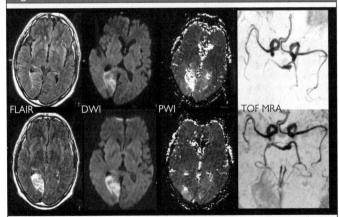

Characterization of stroke using different MRI techniques: upper row – Acute ischaemia in the right posterior cerebral artery territory visible on DWI with slight T2 correlate on FLAIR images. Underlying obstruction in the right posterior cerebral artery is demonstrated on MRA with corresponding hypoperfusion of the complete right posterior cerebral artery territory. Bottom row: On Follow-up MRI the lesion is hyperintense on T2. Along with vessel recanalization perfusion abnormality is largely reduced in size.

Fig 8.6 Susceptibility-weighted T2* MRI.

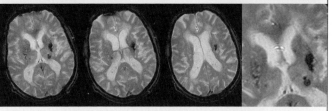

Susceptibility-weighted T2* MRI shows hypointense signal in the left nucleus caudate and thalamus. These microbleeds reflect residual blood, e.g. in haemorrhagic lacunar lesions.

of hypointense signal in T2*-weighted images in projection to the site of vessel occlusion in ischaemic stroke has also been described. In patients with CVT T2* can be useful to visualize hypo-intensities in large veins considered to be correlates of intravenous clots.

8.2.4 **Magnetic resonance angiography**

Magnetic resonance angiography (MRA) is an emerging technique taking advantage of the differences of spin-signals of flowing blood and static tissue, with the stationary tissue signal effectively suppressed relative to the blood flow signal. A single measurement is performed within a few minutes. Two techniques are most widely used to assess narrowing of the extracranial vessels and to visualize the intracranial vasculature: Contrast enhanced MRA (CE-MRA) and time-of-flight (TOF) techniques. MRA source images are frequently post-processed to provide a 3D visualization with an algorithm also termed maximum intensity projection (MIP, see Figure 8.7). This allows the demonstration of 3D vessel topography and offers the possibility to review the vessels in every desirable plane even after the investigation is concluded.

Fig 8.7 MIP Projection of TOF MR-angiography.

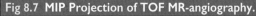
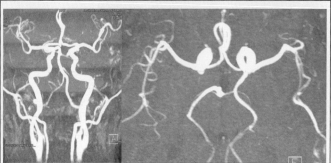

Visualization of the cerebral extra- and intracranial arteries with TOF MR-angiography in multiple, selected planes.

Fig 8.8 Arterial spin labelling MRI techniques (see also Plate 3).

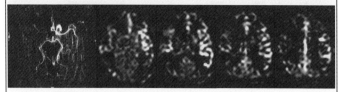

The colour-coded dynamic angiography map (left) describes the time point of maximum blood inflow to arterial vessels; warm colours (red and yellow) indicate early arrival of blood, whereas cold colours (green and blue) indicate later arrival. The figure shows an earlier arrival in the ipsilateral P1 segment and in the contralateral siphon in a patient with a right ICA occlusion. ASL perfusion maps show hypoperfusion in the right MCA territory.

The *ESO Guidelines* recommend the following brain and vascular imaging:

• In patients with suspected transient ischaemic attacks (TIA) or stroke, urgent cranial CT (Class I), or alternatively MRI (Class II), is recommended (Level A)

• If MRI is used, the inclusion of DWI and T2*-weighted gradient echo sequences is recommended (Class II, Level A)

• In patients with TIA, minor stroke or early spontaneous recovery, immediate diagnostic work-up, including urgent vascular imaging (ultrasound, CT angiography, or MR angiography), is recommended (Class I, Level A)

8.2.5 Arterial spin labelling

Arterial spin labelling (ASL) is an MR technique that allows the non-invasive visualization of blood inflow to arterial vessels at several time points after magnetic labelling of a blood bolus. ASL uses magnetization of in-flowing arterial water protons that flow through the vascular tree and exchange magnetization with the unlabelled tissue water. The inflow of magnetically labelled blood to the intracranial circulation can be analysed to obtain subsequent images yielding information about the CBF. Two different applications of ASL are currently available: perfusion maps estimating CBF and bolus arrival time of blood in the cerebral microcirculation, and dynamic ASL angiography providing time-resolved images of blood inflow into large arterial vessels of the circle of Willis (see Figure 8.8).

8.3 Ultrasound imaging in acute stroke

Vascular imaging includes ultrasound and computed tomographic angiography (CTA) or magnetic resonance angiography (MRA) techniques, all of which need appropriate technical equipment, trained investigators and at least some cooperation from the patient.

Specific settings in different hospitals and at different times of the day or week may determine which procedure is used. Studies should be performed as early as possible, but at present they are not needed for fast treatment decisions (although they may be helpful).

8.3.1 Doppler and duplex ultrasound

Doppler and duplex US is best used for rapid detection of extracranial severe obstructive lesions and intracranial mechanisms of stroke (local and embolic obstructions) and more recently US perfusion studies. Transcranial Doppler and duplex use the Doppler effect to measure the direction and velocity of blood flow in the brain (see Figure 8.9). Both methods can also describe intracranial collateral patterns in the presence of extra intracranial embolism, stenoses and occlusion of intracranial vessels, and their spontaneous or therapeutic recanalization.

8.3.2 High intensity transient signals

Using TCD it is possible to detect and count cerebral micro-emboli in intracranial vessels. The principle of the technique is that an embolus backscatters more ultrasonic power than the equivalent volume of blood that it displaces. It therefore produces a transient and short (8–80msec) uni-directional high-intensity signal within the Doppler flow spectrum as shown in Figure 8.10 accompanied by an audible sound, termed high intensity transient signal (HITS) or micro-embolic signal (MES). Micro-emboli monitoring should be a part of routine investigations in stroke patients as these data suggest it might be useful to identify a group of patients who are at risk of recurrent stroke and are most likely to benefit from treatment. Probably MES are associated with a higher stroke risk in patients with asymptomatic carotid stenosis. We suggest not only a sufficiently long monitoring examination (at least 30min), but also repeat examinations in particular once the degree of stenosis progresses.

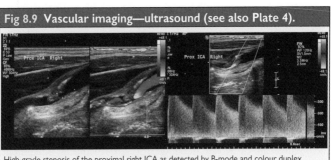

Fig 8.9 Vascular imaging—ultrasound (see also Plate 4).

High-grade stenosis of the proximal right ICA as detected by B-mode and colour duplex ultrasound imaging.

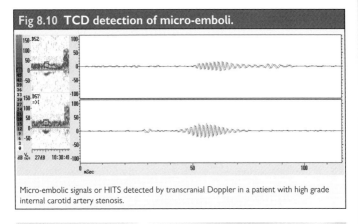

Fig 8.10 TCD detection of micro-emboli.

Micro-embolic signals or HITS detected by transcranial Doppler in a patient with high grade internal carotid artery stenosis.

8.4 Intra-arterial catheter angiography

Intra-arterial catheter angiography has been replaced by the afore-mentioned techniques in patients with ischaemic and often in haemor-rhagic stroke as well. However, it is still the gold standard to identify or exclude intracranial aneurysms in patients with SAH (see Figure 8.11) and often in those with secondary intracranial bleedings sus-pected to be due to AV-malformations. Today, interventional intra-arterial treatment becomes increasingly important and may be applied to patients with ischaemic stroke from intracranial arterial obstruc-tions (stenting, angioplasty), acute thrombo-embolism (intra-arterial thrombolysis and thrombo-embolectomy procedures) (see Chapter 11), as well as in patients with intracranial aneurysms who need pri-mary coiling after SAH.

8.5 Imaging of intracerebral haemorrhage

Acute intracerebral haemorrhage shows an increased attenuation on CT, which is addressed to the high electron density of the pro-tein in haemoglobin. Initially, the increased attenuation is 80–86 Hounsfield units (HU) for up to three days, and then decreases at a rate of 1.5HU/day. Therefore, after around 3 weeks, the haematoma is similar in attenuation to the unaffected brain. In the following early chronic state, the haematoma turns to low, CSF-like attenuation. According to the biochemical evolution of haemorrhages (oxyhae-moglobin → deoxyhaemoglobin → methaemoglobin → haemosid-erin), the signal intensities in MRI compared with the adjacent brain tissue (grey matter) change from similar or low in acute, high in subacute, and low in chronic state in T1-weighted image, or high in hyperacute, low in acute and early subacute, high in late subacute, and low in chronic state in T2-weighted image (see Figure 8.12).

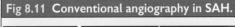

Fig 8.11 Conventional angiography in SAH.

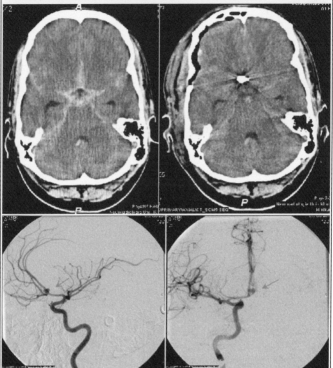

Upper row (left): CT showing hyperdense signal of subarachnoid haemorrhage in the peripontine, basal and posterior fossa cisterns, as well as in the interhemispheric and Sylvian fissures. Bottom row: Conventional angiography showing saccular aneurysm of the ACA in different projections. Upper row right: Post surgery CT showing the location of the clip.

Fig 8.12 MR imaging of acute intracerebral haemorrhage.

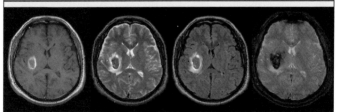

T1-, T2-, T2-weighted FLAIR, and T2*-weighted MRI of a hypertensive intracerebral haemorrhage in the right lateral basal ganglia.

In most patients with a history of arterial hypertension and a typical haematoma location within the basal ganglia, pons or cerebellum, a standard CT is sufficient. If there is no history of arterial hypertension, and if the haemorrhage is atypically located, further diagnostic steps are warranted. Contrast-enhanced CT and CTA can detect many conditions, such as venous sinus thrombosis or large vascular malformations, with a sensitivity that is frequently sufficient, at least for the initial work-up. However, in many patients MRI or conventional angiography is necessary to securely exclude conditions that need immediate treatment. Non-enhanced CT scanning may fail to detect SAH, therefore in case of a typical clinical presentation a lumbar puncture is mandatory. Cranial MRI, combined with MR-venography allows the rapid diagnosis of CVT. Furthermore, changes of the clot signal intensities in MRI show the state of CVT; hence, the duration and dynamic of CVT can be estimated. Conventional cerebral angiography is recommended for all patients with spontaneous intracerebral haemorrhage, except for those older than 45yrs with pre-existing hypertension in thalamic, putaminal, or posterior fossa haemorrhage. Cerebral angiography can detect arterial and venous stenosis, vascular malformations or tumours. Moreover, conventional angiography is urgently indicated when an aneurysm is suspected. Microbleeds are defined as millimetre-sized, $T2^*$ hypointense brain areas representing not only recent, but also past microhaemorrhages, caused by rupture of small blood vessels in subcortical brain tissue, which most often remain clinically asymptomatic. Factors influencing the presence of cerebral microbleeds are age, coexisting small vessel disease with both white matter lesions and lacunar infarctions, as well as CAA. Current data suggests that the risk of haemorrhage attributable to microbleeds after thrombolysis is small and unlikely to exceed the benefits of thrombolytic therapy.

References

Adams Hj, Del Zoppo G, von Kummer R. (2002) *Imaging of the brain and blood vessels in stroke.* 2nd edn. Professional Communications, Inc.

Förster A, Gass A, Kern R, Wolf ME, Hennerici MG, Szabo K. (2011) MRI-guided intravenous thrombolysis in posterior cerebral artery stroke. *Am J Neuroradiol* **32**, 419–21.

Knauth M, von Kummer R, Jansen O, et al. (1997) Potential of CT angiography in acute ischaemic stroke. *Am J Neuroradiol* **18**, 1001–10.

Markus HS, King A, Shipley M, et al. (2010) Asymptomatic embolisation for prediction of stroke in the Asymptomatic Carotid Emboli Study (ACES): a prospective observational study. *Lancet Neurol* **9**, 663–71.

Parizel PM, Makkat S, Van Miert E, et al. (2001) Intracranial haemorrhage: principles of CT and MRI interpretation. *Eur Radiol* **11**, 1770–83.

Ruszkowski J, Damadian R, Giambalvo A, et al. (1986) MRI angiography of the carotid artery. *Magn Reson Imaging* **4**, 497–502.

Sallustio F, Kern R, Günther M, Szabo K, Griebe M, Meairs S, Hennerici M, Gass A, . (2008) Assessment of intracranial collateral flow by using dynamic arterial spin labeling MRA and transcranial color-coded duplex ultrasound. *Stroke* **39**, 1894–1897.

Szabo K, Kern R, Hennerici MG. (2007) Recent advances in imaging in management of symptomatic internal carotid artery disease. *Int J Stroke* **2**, 97–103.

Warach S, Gaa J, Siewert B, et al. (1995) Acute human stroke studied by whole brain echo planar diffusion-weighted MRI. *Ann Neurol* **37**, 231–41.

Zhu XL, Chan MS, Poon WS. (1997) Spontaneous intracranial haemorrhage: which patients need diagnostic cerebral angiography? A prospective study of 206 cases and review of the literature. *Stroke* **28**, 1406–9.

Chapter 9

Stroke subtype classification

> ## Key points
> - Stroke is a heterogeneous disease, therefore careful subtyping is important for research as well as every-day clinical practice.
> - Results of the different diagnostic tests as well as clinical history and presentation have to be considered to determine the most likely aetiology in the individual patient.
> - The recently proposed ASCO system is a complete 'stroke phenotyping' classification as distinguished from past classifications that subtype strokes by characterizing only the most likely cause(s) of stroke.

Subtyping ischaemic stroke can have different purposes, e.g. describing patients' characteristics in a clinical trial, grouping patients in an epidemiological study, careful phenotyping of patients in a genetic study, and very importantly classifying patients for therapeutic decision-making in daily practice. Stroke is a heterogeneous disease with more than 150 known causes (see Table 9.1). Therefore, determining the subtype might be difficult in some cases. Results of the different diagnostic tests, as well as clinical history and presentation have to be considered and taken together to determine the most likely aetiology influencing specific therapy and individual secondary prophylaxis.

9.1 The TOAST classification

Since 1993, most clinical researchers use the classification proposed by the Trial of ORG 10172 in Acute Stroke Treatment (TOAST) investigators. The original purpose of this classification was to better characterize the TOAST cohort of patients in order to investigate the potential efficacy of danaparoid in various stroke subtypes. The TOAST investigators defined 11 categories of stroke,

Table 9.1 Stroke subtypes

1. *Ischaemic*
1.1 Large vessel disease
1.1.1 Extracranial
1.1.2 Intracranial
1.2 Small vessel disease
1.3 Cardiac emboli
1.4 Other causes
1.4.1 Dissection
1.4.2 Rare or hereditary large- or medium-sized artery disease
(e.g. Moya-moya disease, fibromuscular dysplasia)
1.4.3 Rare or hereditary small vessel disease
1.4.4 Coagulopathy
1.4.5 Metabolic disease with arteriopathy
1.4.6 Vasculitis
1.4.7 Other rare entities
1.5 Co-existing causes
1.6 Unknown
1.7 Unclassifiable

2. *Haemorrhagic*
2.1 Hypertension-related small vessel disease (haemorrhagic type)
2.2 Cerebral amyloid angiopathy
2.2.1 Sporadic
2.2.2 Hereditary
2.3 Bleeding diathesis
2.3.1 Drugs that decrease clotting
2.3.2 Other haemostatic or hematologic disorders
2.4 Vascular malformation
2.4.1 Arteriovenous malformation
2.4.2 Dural fistula
2.4.3 Ruptured aneurysm
2.4.4 Cavernoma
2.4.4.1 Sporadic
2.4.4.2 Familial
2.5 Other causes
2.5.1 Tumour-related
2.5.2 Toxic (e.g. sympathomimetic drugs, cocaine)
2.5.3 Trauma
2.5.4 Arteritis, angiitis, endocarditis (ruptured mycotic aneurysm), infections
2.5.5 Rare entities (e.g. dissection of intracranial arteries)
2.6 Co-existing cause
2.7 Unknown
2.8 Unclassifiable

3. *Subarachnoid haemorrhage*
3.1 With aneurysm
3.2 With dissection

3.3 Traumatic

3.4 Neoplastic (melanoma)

3.5 Unknown

4. *Cerebral venous thrombosis*

5. *Spinal cord stroke*

5.1 Ischaemic

5.2 Haemorrhagic

5.2.1 Associated with arteriovenous malformation

5.2.2 Associated with coagulopathy

which were subdivided into five groups (Table 9.2). Only these five groups were used in further clinical research. However, weaknesses of the TOAST classification are that in the study nearly 40% of ischaemic stroke remained of "undetermined/unclassified" aetiology and evaluation was mainly CT-based.

9.2 Stroke Data Bank subtype classification

Derived from the Harvard Stroke Registry classification, the National Institute of Neurological Disorders and Stroke (NINDS) Stroke Data Bank recognized five major groups: brain haemorrhages; brain infarctions, and among them atherothrombotic and tandem arterial pathological abnormalities; cardio-embolic stroke; lacunar stroke; and stroke from rare causes or undetermined aetiology (Table 9.3). Weaknesses of this classification include the very restrictive definition for atherothrombotic stroke and the wide definition of lacunar strokes.

Table 9.2 Modified TOAST classification of ischaemic stroke subtypes

1. Large-artery atherosclerosis	– >50% stenosis or occlusion of a major brain artery – No cardiac source of embolism – No subcortical or brainstem infarct <1.5cm
2. Cardio-embolism	– High- and medium-risk aetiologies defined
3. Small vessel occlusion	– Clinical lacunar syndrome – History of diabetes and hypertension – Lesion <1.5cm
4. Stroke of other determined cause	– Non-atherosclerotic vasculopathies, hyper-coagulable states, hematologic disorders
5. Stroke of undetermined cause	– Two or more causes defined – Negative or incomplete evaluation

99

Table 9.3 NINDS-Stroke Data Bank subtype classification

Atherothrombosis	– 90% stenosis or occlusion on angiography of the internal carotid artery origin or siphon, basilar artery or major cerebral artery stem – Tandem arterial pathology
Cardiac embolism	– Cardiac source recognized
Lacune	– Clinical lacunar syndrome – Small deep infarct on CT or normal CT after 1 week – Normal angiography
Unusual causes	– Arteriitis, dissection, fibromuscular dysplasia, sickle cell anaemia – Stroke in migraine or mycotic aneurysm – Other rare or unusual cause
Infarction of unde-termined cause	– This was replaced eventually by the term *cryptogenic stroke*

9.3 Oxfordshire Community Stroke Project subtype classification

The classification from the Oxfordshire Community Stroke Project (OCSP) was proposed to characterize this population-based epidemiological study. The investigators had to cope with the quality and cost of the workup available at that time in the UK. Transient ischaemic attacks (TIA) and strokes were detected and investigated by general practitioners. The classification was based on clinical findings only. Computed tomography (CT) scanning was the only investigational test performed; assessment of extra- and intracranial arteries and precise cardiac work-up were not available. This probably led the OCSP investigators to classify patients according to the extent and site of brain infarction on clinical grounds alone (Table 9.4).

Table 9.4 Oxfordshire Community Stroke project subtype classification

1. Cerebral infarct	– CT diagnosis within 28 days or post–mortem
2. LACI – lacunar infarcts	– One of the 4 clinical lacunar syndromes
3. TACI – total anterior circulation infarcts	– New higher cerebral dysfunction plus ipsilateral motor and/or sensory deficit of 2 areas (face, arm, or leg)
4. PACI – partial anterior circulation infarcts	– Only 2 of the 3 components of the TACI syndrome
5. POCI – posterior circulation infarcts	– Defined posterior circulation syndrome

Fig 9.1 Example for the ASCO classification system.

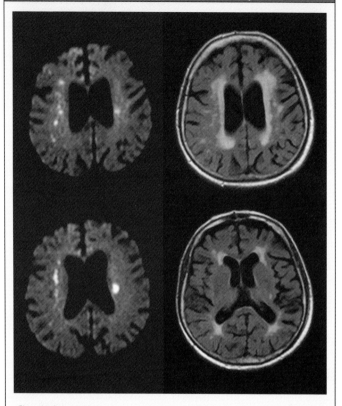

Clinical information:

- 90 year-old woman
- Acute onset of right hemiparesis
- History of paroxysmal atrial fibrillation
- Work-up: 80% stenosis of the right internal carotid artery
- MRI: bi-hemispheric acute ischaemic stroke (L lacunar, R haemodynamic pattern); leukoaraiosis

TOAST Classification **undetermined cause of stroke:**

- Cardiac cause (AF) + large vessel disease (symptomatic carotid stenosis)

ASCO Classification **A1 S1 C3 O0:**

- A1 (symptomatic carotid stenosis with high evidence)
- S1 (lacunar infarction + severe SVD with high evidence)
- C3 (atrial fibrillation with low evidence of stroke relationship)
- O0 (no other cause)

9.4 **The A-S-C-O (phenotypic) classification of stroke**

This new approach to stroke subtyping was proposed only recently. The concept is to introduce an evidence-based 'stroke phenotyping' classification (i.e. stroke aetiology and the presence of all underlying diseases, divided by grade of likelihood as source of individual stroke) as distinguished from past classifications that subtype strokes by characterizing only the most likely cause(s) of stroke. In this phenotype-based classification, every patient is characterized by A-S-C-O: A for atherosclerosis, S for small vessel disease, C for cardiac source, O for other cause. Each of the 4 phenotypes is graded 1–3, where 1 is 'definitely a potential cause of the index stroke', 2 is 'causality uncertain', and 3 is 'unlikely a direct cause of the index stroke (but disease is present)'. When the disease is completely absent, the grade is 0; when grading is not possible due to insufficient work-up, the grade is 9.

With this new way of classifying patients, no information is neglected when the diagnosis is made, treatment can be adapted to the observed phenotypes and the most likely aetiology (e.g. grade 1 in 1 of the 4 A-S-C-O phenotypes, see Figure 9.1), and analyses in clinical research can be based on one of the four phenotypes (e.g. for genetic analysis purpose), while clinical trials can focus on one or several of these four phenotypes (e.g. focus on patients A1-A2-A3).

References

Adams HP, Bendixen BH, Kappelle LJ, et al. (1993) Classification of subtype of acute ischemic stroke: definitions for use in a multicenter clinical trial. *Stroke* **24**, 35–41.

Amarenco P, Bogousslavsky J, Caplan LR, Donnan GA, Hennerici MG. (2009) Classification of stroke subtypes. *Cerebrovasc Dis* **27,** 493–501.

Amarenco P, Bogousslavsky J, Caplan LR, Donnan GA, Hennerici MG. (2009) New approach to stroke subtyping: the A-S-C-O (phenotypic) classification of stroke. *Cerebrovascular Dis* **27**, 502–8.

Bamford J, Sandercock PA, Dennis MS, Burn J, Warlow CP. (1991) Classification and natural history of clinically identifiable subtypes of brain infarction. *Lancet* **337**, 1521–6.

Landau WM, Nassief A. (2005) Time to burn the TOAST. *Stroke* **36**, 902–4.

Lindley RI, Warlow CP, Wardlaw JM, Dennis MS, Slattery J, Sandercock PA. (1993) Interobserver reliability of a clinical classification of acute cerebral infarction. *Stroke* **24**, 1801–4.

Mohr JP, Caplan LR, Melski JW, et al. (1978) The Harvard Cooperative Stroke Registry: a prospective registry. *Neurology* **28**, 754–62.

Acute stroke management and treatment

Chapter 10

Management of acute stroke

Key points

- Due to the short time window for specific treatment of acute stroke, fast and well co-ordinated emergency management is essential for further prognosis.
- Beyond the beneficial effects of thrombolysis, a treatment on a stroke unit is associated with a significant and long-lasting reduction of mortality and morbidity.
- General management on a stroke unit includes respiratory and cardiac care, fluid and serum glucose management, blood pressure control, prevention and treatment of seizures, aspiration, fever, infections, pressure ulcers, depression, agitation and falls.
- Early rehabilitation measures may prevent complications related to immobilization and seem safe and feasible.

10.1 Public awareness and pre-hospital management

10.1.1 Public awareness and education

Because of the vulnerability of neurons a rapid and specific therapy for acute stroke is essential for both early improvement and long-term favourable clinical outcome. Therefore, it is very important that management at all stages of acute stroke care is effective in time and processes to avoid any delay (Figure 10.1). This includes a broad public awareness of stroke (i.e. that stroke signs should be noticed by patients and their relatives, and trigger calling the ambulance), pre-hospital first aid by emergency services, and also in-hospital management. Effectiveness at all stages of acute stroke needs to be realized by public campaigns mediating stroke signs and the burden

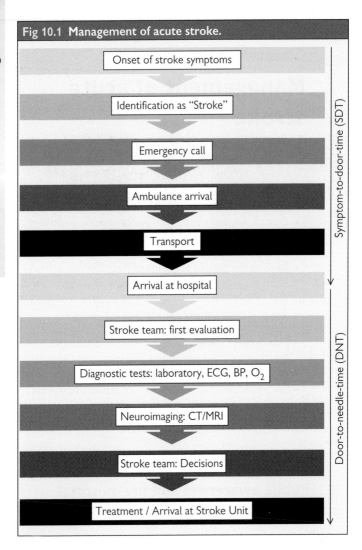

Fig 10.1 Management of acute stroke.

Onset of stroke symptoms

Identification as "Stroke"

Emergency call

Ambulance arrival

Transport

Arrival at hospital

Stroke team: first evaluation

Diagnostic tests: laboratory, ECG, BP, O₂

Neuroimaging: CT/MRI

Stroke team: Decisions

Treatment / Arrival at Stroke Unit

Symptom-to-door-time (SDT)

Door-to-needle-time (DNT)

of stroke, and by systematic and continuous education of pre- and in-hospital caregivers.

Beyond the urgent need for educational programmes regarding healthy lifestyle for primary prevention of stroke, there is a similar need to increase the awareness in the population about stroke signs, their sometimes initially transient character, and early therapy options ('time is brain' concept). Educational programmes directed at the public are served via mass media, general practitioners, and friends and relatives. Several studies on such programmes showed

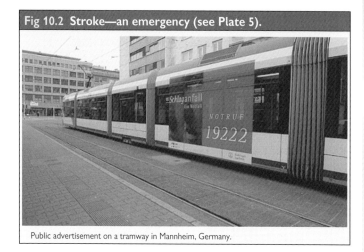

Fig 10.2 **Stroke—an emergency (see Plate 5).**

Public advertisement on a tramway in Mannheim, Germany.

positive effects on the pre-hospital time delay, but these effects decrease after termination of the educational programmes. These findings emphasize the importance of continuous public education to sustain stroke awareness in the population (Figure 10.2).

10.1.2 **Pre-hospital care**

Since it is not possible to differentiate ischaemic stroke from intracranial haemorrhage on clinical grounds alone (signs and symptoms), it is necessary to immediately transport the patient to a department where neuroimaging can be performed. Emergency services have to identify suspected stroke victims accurately and assure an immediate transfer to the nearest hospital with a stroke unit. Emergency services should notify the hospital in advance in order to prompt immediate preparation. As suggested by several studies, pre-notification of the hospital reduces in-hospital delay, increases the time window for thrombolytic treatment and improves outcome. Systematic training programmes for paramedics improve clinical skills and knowledge of stroke symptoms (including widely used scores, e.g. GCS, NIHSS, FAST), and therefore decrease pre-hospital delays.

Before transport, vital signs, including blood pressure, respiratory function, and serum glucose, need to be assessed. 2–4L/min of supplemental oxygen via a nasal tube are generally recommended. A large intravenous access should be placed and isotonic saline solution given intravenously. Although not very common in acute stroke, the patient may require intubation and ventilation in cases of respiratory failure. A brief neurological examination should be performed including Glasgow Coma Score (GCS); this is particularly important if intubation is required, since neurological functions will be difficult to judge thereafter (Table 10.1).

Table 10.1 Pre-hospital management of acute stroke
Pre-hospital management of acute stroke: 'not-to-do rules'
Don't give aspirin or heparin before diagnosis and treatment decisions
Avoid hypotension or abrupt drops of blood pressure—The blood pressure should only be lowered carefully if above 220 systolic and/or 120mmHg diastolic at repeated measurements
Don't do any intraarterial or intramuscular injections or punctures
Don't give any oral nutrition; keep the patient fasting to prevent aspiration
Don't give the patient glucose or other hypotonic solutions iv

During transport, the vital signs—airways, breathing, and circulation—need to be monitored continuously. Transport should be immediate and as fast as possible, thus lights and sirens must be used, and the nearest specialist hospital should be headed for that offers an expert stroke service with 24hr, 7 days a week access to neuroimaging and neurological care. Helicopter use may be considered for remote areas for patients within the time window.

Emergency medical services should carefully ask for the exact time of stroke symptom onset. One of the most common mistakes is to confuse the 'time of symptom onset' with the 'time last seen normal' if stroke symptoms occurred unobserved. Medication—in particular anticoagulation, larger operations in the recent past, and relevant concomitant disease should be documented. To take a witness, or at least his or her phone number, will help the physician in the hospital to answer further questions later.

10.2 **In-hospital management**

10.2.1 **Emergency department**

After arrival in the hospital and handing the patient over to the stroke team, a first evaluation is made in the emergency department: Vital signs need to be checked, and, if stable, a brief medical history and neurological examination is performed. The exact time of onset should be reassessed at this stage. After assessment of the stroke syndrome and its acuity, a process of further diagnostics, including laboratory tests, echocardiography (ECG), and neuroimaging have to be realized. When the result of brain imaging is available, a treatment decision can be made by the stroke team and the patient will be transferred to the stroke unit. The time interval between arrival at the hospital and start of treatment is referred to as 'door to needle time'. Recommendations suggest that patients should be seen and examined clinically within 15min. Neuroimaging should be done within 25–30min, with the result being available after 45min. Treatment should start no later than 60min after arrival in the hospital. In the Safe Implementation of Thrombolysis in Stroke-Monitoring Study (SITS-MOST), however, the mean door-to-needle time was 68min and only 10.6% of tissue plaminogen activator (alteplase)-treated patients received the therapy within 90 min after onset.

Various reasons may contribute to in-hospital delays. Symptoms might not be recognized as an emergency by the medical staff and the patient may therefore be seen too late by the stroke physician. In-hospital transport may be inefficient, or there can be delays related to neuroimaging or laboratory test capacities. Organized stroke care pathways are useful and a written stroke care protocol should be available. 'Door-to-imaging' and 'door-to-needle' times need to be monitored continuously. Acute stroke patients should be triaged in the emergency department with the same priority as patients with myocardial infarction, and patients eligible for thrombolysis require priority for computed tomography (CT). Delays after neuroimaging can be avoided by starting thrombolysis early thereafter, for example, in the vicinity of CT or in the emergency department.

10.2.2 Stroke Unit: concept and principles

A specialized stroke unit is defined as a 'hospital unit that exclusively takes care of stroke patients with specially trained staff and a multidisciplinary approach to treatment and care' (Table 10.2). Treatment on a stroke unit is associated with a better outcome in mortality and

Table 10.2 ESO recommendations for stroke management

ESO recommendations: admission to stroke units

1. Stroke patients should be treated in stroke units
2. Stroke units have to provide co-ordinated multidisciplinary care given by medical, nursing and therapy staff who specialize in stroke care
3. Patients with subarachnoid haemorrhage should be referred to stroke units with facilities for neurosurgical treatment, neuroradiological interventions, and neuro-intensive care

ESO recommendations: patient management on stroke units

1. Stabilize the patient's general condition
2. Give therapy directed at specific aspects of stroke pathogenesis (e.g. recanalization of vessel occlusion or a prevention of mechanisms leading to neuronal death)
3. Treat complications (such as secondary haemorrhage, space occupying oedema, seizures, aspiration, infection, decubital ulcers, deep venous thrombosis, or pulmonary embolism)
4. Initiate early secondary prevention measures to reduce the incidence of stroke recurrence
5. Begin rehabilitation measures

disability, and with a long-lasting benefit compared with treatment on a general medical ward. Although stroke unit care is more expensive than treatment on general medical wards, it reduces overall in-patient care costs and is cost-effective. Immediate care should not be restricted to patients eligible for alteplase therapy, since the benefit on morbidity and mortality is independent from the beneficial effects of alteplase.

During treatment on the stroke unit regular clinical visits during and after acute therapy by a multidisciplinary team (neurologists, internists, stroke nurses, physiotherapists, occupational therapists, speech therapists, neuropsychologist) including regular assessment of the clinical and neurological status (e.g. NIHSS scores) is necessary. Written care protocols for acute stroke patients should be available. Implementing a continuous quality improvement scheme can also diminish in-hospital delays. Benchmarks should be defined and measured for individual institutions. They have recently been developed for regional networks and countries. Regular quality control of managements in standardized protocols is requested by health authorities in several countries in Europe.

Medical treatment on the stroke unit includes thrombolysis with alteplase and other specific acute therapies, but also early secondary prevention. This is very important due to the high early stroke recurrence rates of up to 20% within the first week after TIA or stroke. Other medical aspects of stroke unit care are the treatment of prolonged stroke symptoms (i.e. disturbed consciousness, aphasia, dysphagia, paresis, etc.), and the prevention or treatment of early complications (e.g. fever, aspiration pneumonia, urinary tract infection, post-stroke depression, etc.). A complete diagnostic work-up needs to be carried out to identify treatable causes for immediate secondary prevention (e.g. symptomatic large artery disease, cardiac sources of embolism).

Clinical symptoms predicting later stroke-related complications, and medical conditions such as hypertensive crisis, aspiration pneumonia, and cardiac or renal failure, have to be recognized as early as possible. These signs can be recorded by continuous monitoring of vital parameters (ECG and blood pressure monitoring, arterial oxygen saturation using infrared pulse oxymetry, respiration frequency, body temperature, and serum glucose), clinical examination of cardiac and pulmonary function, evaluation of concomitant heart disease, and assessment of early signs of dysphagia.

10.3 **Diagnostic procedures**

The diagnostic procedures during early management of stroke can be divided into two parts: first-line (emergency) diagnostic procedures, which focus on decision making for thrombolysis and for other acute treatment options; and second-line (elective) diagnostic procedures that focus on the individual risk profile of each patient as a basis for an effective secondary prevention.

The *ESO Guidelines* recommend the following diagnostic work-up:

- In patients with acute stroke and TIA, early clinical evaluation, including physiological parameters and routine blood tests, is recommended (Class I, Level A)
- For all stroke and TIA patients, a sequence of blood tests is recommended (see Table 10.3 below)
- It is recommended that all acute stroke and TIA patients should have a 12-lead ECG. In addition, continuous ECG recording is recommended for ischaemic stroke and TIA patients (Class I, Level A)
- It is recommended that for stroke and TIA patients seen after the acute phase, 24-h Holter ECG monitoring should be performed when arrhythmias are suspected and no other causes of stroke are found (Class I, Level A)
- Echocardiography is recommended in selected patients (Class III, Level B)

Table 10.3 Subsequent laboratory tests, according to the type of stroke and suspected aetiology

All patients	Full blood count, electrolytes, glucose, lipids, creatinine, CRP, or ESR
Cerebral venous thrombosis, hypercoagulopathy	Thrombophilia screen, AT3, Factor 2, 5, mutations, factor 8, protein C, protein S, antiphospholipid-antibodies, d-dimer, homocysteine
Bleeding disorder	INR, aPTT, fibrinogen, etc.
Vascular or systemic disorder	Cerebral spinal fluid, auto-antibody screen, specific antibodies or PCR for HIV, syphilis, borreliosis, tuberculosis, fungi, illicit drug- screening, blood culture
Suspected genetic disorders, e.g. mitochondrial disorders (MELAS), CADASIL, sickle cell disease, Fabry disease, multiple cavernoma, etc.	Specific tests

The selection of the appropriate diagnostic procedures has to be based on clinical and neurological evaluation. Patients' medical and surgical history (medication, prior stroke, prior surgical procedures, cardiac pacemakers, etc.) should be considered carefully. Due to the lack of time during the hyperacute phase, a basic, but sufficient physical examination should be performed, including all aspects of respiratory and cardiovascular function.

10.3.1 Brain imaging

In the acute setting, it is very important to decide which brain imaging technique is used. Most centres use non-contrast CT as the standard

Fig 10.3 Emergency CT in acute stroke (see Plate 6).

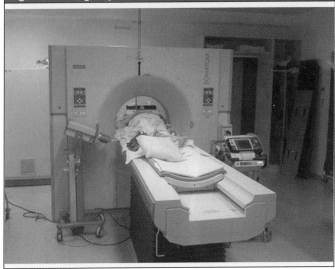

procedure for all stroke patients. CT is fast and can exclude intracranial haemorrhage for treatment decision within the 4.5-hr time window (Figure 10.3). CT may also identify stroke mimics, e.g. a subdural haemorrhage, a brain tumour, or chronic infarction. Although CT angiography and CT perfusion may facilitate treatment decisions, they are not recommended as routine for every patient, since they may have side effects and produce time delays. In cerebral ischaemia CT is mostly negative in the acute phase and has a very poor overall sensitivity in the posterior fossa. Therefore, MRI protocols including DWI, MRA, and perfusion imaging are currently replacing CT as the initial radiological examination in many stroke centres. MRI requires a good infrastructure and dedicated acute stroke protocols. Only then, it may be performed with almost comparable scanning times. MRI is contraindicated in patients with pacemakers, neurostimulators, metal fragments, etc. and can be impossible if co-operation is poor.

10.3.2 **Laboratory investigations**

Several laboratory tests should be performed routinely in patients with suspected acute stroke to identify conditions that may mimic or cause stroke or that may influence therapeutic options. In the emergency room a blood sample has to be taken for immediate laboratory analysis of the following parameters:

- *Coagulation parameters (INR, aPTT)*: Many patients with acute stroke are taking anticoagulants (heparin or warfarin). Thrombolytic therapy treatment decisions require information on coagulation status. An elevated international normalized ratio (INR) may exclude stroke patients from receiving alteplase. Fibrinolytic therapy with alteplase should not be performed in patients treated with other novel anticoagulants such as dabigatran, rivaroxaban, apixaban or edoxaban when plasma levels of anticoagulants are present. As elimination kinetics may vary, depending on renal and hepatic function, body mass and age, measurement of the anticoagulant effect of the drug by functional assays, or measurement of drug levels, must be recommended before attempting alteplase treatment. For direct thrombin inhibitors, thrombin time or related assays provide the most reliable information but at present are still time consuming (approximately 20 min). Similarly, for direct factor Xa inhibitors, antifactor Xa assays (chromogenic assays, but also clotting assays) can be used but require specific calibration, as the conventional calibrators based on low-molecular-weight heparin cannot be used (Dempfle and Hennerici 2011).

- *Complete blood count, including platelets:* A blood cell count provides essential information regarding haemoglobin and haematocrit, as well as platelet count, which is important in candidates for alteplase therapy. Additionally, blood cell abnormalities such as sickle cell disease, polycythaemia, and thrombocytosis increase the risk for stroke.
- *Glucose:* Hypoglycaemia is the most common abnormality that may mimic acute stroke. It is easily corrected with rapid resolution of symptoms. On the other hand, between 25 and 50% of patients with acute ischaemic and haemorrhagic stroke are hyperglycaemic on presentation. Hyperglycaemia has been associated with a worsened outcome due to an increase in the amount of cerebral oedema, a greater likelihood of haemorrhagic transformation in patients treated with alteplase, a longer hospital stay and higher mortality rate.
- *Cardiac enzymes: creatine kinase or troponin:* Not infrequently patients with acute stroke suffer acute myocardial infarction.
- *C-reactive protein:* C-reactive protein (CRP) is one of the acute phase proteins that increase during systemic inflammation. But as recent research suggests an elevated CRP is associated with a higher cardiovascular risk and a worse outcome in patients with ischaemic stroke.
- *Electrolytes:* Electrolyte disorders and uraemia may cause mental and physical deficits mimicking the diagnosis of stroke.
- *Blood gas analysis:* If considering thrombolytics, arterial punctures should be avoided unless absolutely necessary.

Additional laboratory tests are tailored to the individual patient including toxicology screen, lipid profile, sedimentation rate, antinuclear antibody (ANA), rheumatoid factor, and homocysteine. Detailed studies of coagulation factors and coagulation in patients with possible hypercoagulable states, should include protein C, protein S, antithrombin III, and Factor V Leiden testing.

10.3.3 **Other diagnostic procedures**

In all stroke and TIA patients, further diagnostic work-up, including vascular imaging (extracranial and transcranial Doppler/duplex ultrasound, CT-angiography, or MR angiography) and cardiac diagnostics are necessary. Echocardiography should be performed in all patients, but particularly in those with territorial or embolic stroke to reveal any cardio-embolic source (e.g. thrombus in the left atrium or atrial septal aneurysm) or an atheroma in the arch of the aorta. Moreover, an echocardiogram may be useful to detect a shunt from right to left atrium through a patent foramen ovale or atrial septal defect. The accuracy of this ultrasound examination is significantly increased by transoesophageal echocardiography. PFO detection can also be performed with transcranial Doppler ultrasound (TCD) after administration of echocontrast agents or agitated saline solution. CT angiography of the aortic arch is better to identify atherosclerotic plaques at the origin of carotid, innominate and subclavian/vertebral arteries as potential sources for embolism.

10.4 **General treatment of stroke**

General treatment of stroke aims at stabilizing the critically ill patient and is a crucial part of stroke unit care. General treatment includes respiratory and cardiac care, fluid and metabolic management, blood pressure control, prevention and treatment of seizures, early mobilization to prevent venous thrombo-embolism, early assessment of dysphagia and treatment of aspiration, fever, infections, pressure ulcers, depression, agitation, and falls. The control of these factors requires continuous monitoring during the first 24–72hr after admission. However, many aspects of general treatment have not been systematically investigated in randomized studies.

10.4.1 **Respiratory function and dysphagia**

Normal respiratory function and adequate blood oxygenation are essential for stroke management. Respiratory function should be monitored to detect and treat hypoxia (particularly in patients with extensive brainstem or hemispheric infarction, intracranial haemorrhage, or sustained seizure activity) or complications such as severe pneumonia or chronic obstructive pulmonary disease. Blood oxygenation is improved by giving 2–4L/min oxygen via a nasal tube. In the case of severely compromised respiratory function, severe hypoxaemia and hypercarbia, and in the unconscious patient at high risk of aspiration, early intubation may be necessary. Bacterial pneumonia accounts for about 20% of deaths after stroke and may be due to aspiration, failure to clear secretions, and reduced chest wall movement on the hemiparetic side. Aspiration is frequently found in patients with impaired consciousness, impaired gag reflex, and swallowing disturbances. The frequency of clinically-assessed dysphagia in patients with stroke is 35% or more. Appropriate antibiotics should be given early in patients at risk for pulmonary infection.

10.4.2 Cardiac disease and blood pressure

Cardiac care includes monitoring and treatment of severe cardiac arrhythmias, heart failure or acute myocardial infarction. Significant ECG alterations in the ST segments, the T waves and QT prolongation mimicking myocardial ischaemia may appear in the acute phase. Therefore, every stroke patient should have continuous ECG monitoring at least within the first 24hr. Further laboratory analyses including heart enzymes and troponine should be considered. Increased troponine or hs-troponine values should be re-examined: if values increase further, patients should undergo careful cardiological work-up for suspected MI. Optimizing cardiac output by maintaining a high normal blood pressure and a normal heart rate are essential. Increases in cardiac output may increase cerebral perfusion in areas which have lost their autoregulative capacity after acute cerebral ischaemia.

Blood pressure monitoring and treatment during acute stroke management is a matter of controversy, and the current guidelines for management of hypertension are not evidence-based. The present recommendation is to not treat hypertension in most patients with ischaemic stroke, unless blood pressure exceeds 200–220mmHg systolic or 120–140mmHg diastolic. Systemic thrombolysis should only be given if the blood pressure is lower than 185mmHg systolic and 105–110mmHg diastolic. Current guidelines do not support interventions to increase blood pressure in patients with acute ischaemic stroke. Very high blood pressure constitutes an indication for early, but cautious drug treatment avoiding abrupt reduction, because of altered autoregulation of cerebral blood flow in hypertensive patients and the risk of poor perfusion of affected brain area in brisk lowering. There are only a few other indications for immediate antihypertensive therapy (e.g. concomitant myocardial ischaemia, cardiac insufficiency, acute renal failure, and aortic arch dissection). On the other hand, patients with spontaneous intracerebral haemorrhage require immediate intervention if hypertension is present; careful monitoring should control the efficacy of antihypertensive treatment. The use of sublingual nifedipine should be avoided because of the risk of abrupt reduction of blood pressure or overshoot hypertension. Oral captopril may be used instead, but has a short duration of action and can have an abrupt effect. Additionally, intravenous labetalol is frequently recommended and intravenous urapidil is increasingly used.

10.4.3 **Serum glucose**

Hyperglycaemia occurs in up to 60% of stroke patients without known diabetes, and is associated with larger infarcts and with poor functional outcome. There is limited evidence whether reduction of glucose in acute stroke improves prognosis. In most stroke units it is common practice to reduce blood glucose levels exceeding 200mg/dL (11.2mmol/L), intravenous insulin treatment seem to be safe and feasible, but careful monitoring is mandatory to avoid severe hypoglycaemia. Hypoglycaemia below 50mg/dL (2.8mmol/L) may mimic acute stroke, and should be treated by intravenous dextrose bolus or infusion of 10–20% glucose.

Treatment of hyperglycaemia should be started early on, preferably in the same time window as applicable for thrombolysis, targeting salvageable tissue, and sustained for longer periods of time (e.g. 3–5 days). Direct and indirect potential toxic effects of hyperglycaemia are more prominent in larger infarctions. Moreover, patients with lacunar stroke seem to profit from hyperglycaemia up to a concentration of 12mmol/L (216mg/dL). Whether more aggressive regimens of serum glucose reduction can be recommended to achieve levels between 4.5 and 6mmol/L (81–108mg/dL) using intravenous insulin remains unclear since the multi-centre trial NICE-SUGAR showed an increase of the absolute risk of mortality by 2.6% in this group.

10.4.4 **Nutrition, fluid, and electrolytes**

Stroke patients should have a balanced fluid and electrolyte status to avoid plasma volume contraction, which influences brain perfusion and kidney function. Some degree of dehydration on admission is frequent and may be related to bad outcome. Virtually all acute stroke patients need intravenous fluid therapy, with more or less positive balance according to level of dehydration. Uncontrolled volume replacement, however, may lead to cardiac failure and pulmonary oedema. Therefore, a slightly negative fluid balance is recommended in the presence of brain oedema, but hypotonic solutions are contraindicated.

In comatose patients or in patients with dysphagia, nutrition may be provided initially by intravenous solutions, but feeding by a nasogastric tube should be considered when the patient is neurologically stable. If the patient is alert and able to swallow, oral feeding should be started with a liquid or mechanical soft diet, followed by bland or regular diets.

10.4.5 **Fever and infections**

Fever is frequently seen after the onset of stroke and negatively influences clinical outcome. A raised body temperature must initiate a search for infection and adequate treatment. A small number of studies with systematic antipyretic medication failed to shown any benefit, although treatment of raised body temperature above 37.5°C is common practice in stroke patients. Whether hypothermia below 35°C is beneficial to patients with acute stroke as suggested by experimental data will be studied in currently prepared RCTs (EuroHYP). In patients with acute severe stroke, prophylactic administration of antibiotics lowers the rate of infection, avoids increases of body temperature, and may be associated with a better clinical outcome.

10.4.6 Deep vein thrombosis and pulmonary embolism

The risk of deep vein thrombosis and pulmonary embolism can be reduced by early hydration and early mobilization. In stroke patients low-dose low-molecular-weight heparin reduces the incidence of severe deep vein thrombosis and pulmonary embolism without increasing the risk of intracranial or extracranial haemorrhage. These drugs should be administered in high risk patients (e.g. in patients with history of recent pulmonary embolism). The use of stockings failed to show any significant effect.

10.4.7 Pressure ulcers

As in every critically ill patients stroke patients are at high risk of developing pressure ulcers. The use of support surfaces, frequent repositioning, and care of sacral skin are adequate preventive strategies, as well as appropriate nursing of incontinent patients. For patients at high risk, pressure-relieving devices, like foam theatre mattress or air-filled mattress systems, should be used.

10.4.8 Incontinence and urinary tract infections

Urinary incontinence is common after stroke due to disturbance of central bladder function. Studies suggest a prevalence of 40–60% early after acute stroke, with 25% still incontinent at discharge and 15% remaining chronically incontinent. Structured assessment and physical management have been shown to improve continence rates in both inpatients and outpatients. The majority of hospital-acquired urinary tract infections are associated with the use of indwelling catheters and should therefore be avoided if possible. Once urinary infection is diagnosed, appropriate antibiotics should be chosen to prevent fever and systemic infection.

10.4.9 Seizures

Focal and secondary generalized seizures may occur at onset or in the acute phase of ischaemic stroke. In contrast to approval regulations, the ESO and the AHA recommendations state that, a patient with a seizure at the time of onset of stroke may be eligible for treatment with alteplase as long as the physician is convinced that residual impairments are secondary to stroke and not a postictal phenomenon

(Class IIa, Level of Evidence C). This recommendation differs from the previous statements and represents a broadening of eligibility for treatment with alteplase. Post-stroke epilepsy may develop in 3–4% of patients. The risk of having an epileptic seizure is higher in patients with large ischaemic strokes involving the cortex with small areas of preserved 'cortical islands'. Standard anti-epileptic drugs should be used based on general principles of seizure management. Prophylactic administration of anticonvulsant drugs to patients with recent stroke who have not had seizures is not recommended.

10.4.10 **Neuropsychiatric complications**

Agitation and confusion may be caused by acute stroke, but more frequently are a symptom of other complications such as fever, volume depletion or infection. Adequate treatment of the underlying cause must precede any type of sedation or antipsychotic treatment. Cognitive deficits and depression are frequent complications of stroke and affect approximately 60–75% of all survivors. Severe depression occurs in approximately one-third of all patients after stroke with highest risks if lesions were located in the frontal lobe of the dominant hemisphere. Stroke physicians should be aware of the relevance of post stroke depression; psychotherapy and/or antidepressant drugs should therefore be considered.

Sleep-wake disturbances are also more common than hitherto believed and may affect stroke outcome. Sleep-wake disturbances including insomnia, disturbances of wakefulness (hypersomnia, excessive daytime sleepiness, fatigue), sleep-related movement disorders (restless legs syndrome, periodic limb movements during sleep), and parasomnias REM sleep behaviour disorder) are found in 10–50% of patients.

10.5 **Early rehabilitation measures**

Early rehabilitation measures by a multi-disciplinary team belong to the fundamental components of stroke unit care. Early mobilization is important to avoid secondary complications such as thrombo-embolism, pneumonia, and pressure ulceration. However, no randomized clinical trial has shown significant effects on death and dependency by early mobilization. The optimal timing to start rehabilitation measures in acute stroke is unclear. Data from experimental studies (functional neuroimaging and animal studies) define the peri-infarct period as the crucial time to begin rehabilitation. Trials comparing "early" and "late" initiation of rehabilitation have reported controversial results, some suggesting improved prognosis if therapy is started within 20–30 days. The optimal timing of first mobilization is unclear, but results from the AVERT study suggested that immediate physical therapy within 24hr is safe, well tolerated, feasible and beneficial. Early rehabilitation measures, especially focusing on activities of daily living, need a multidisciplinary team. These teams usually consist of stroke physicians, nursing staff, physiotherapists, occupational therapists, speech therapists, and neuropsychologists. Early supported discharge from a stroke unit reduces the length of hospital stay and improves the long-term clinical outcome. Therefore, social services should also be integrated in the multidisciplinary stroke unit team.

References

Adams HP, del Zoppo G, Alberts MJ, et al. (2007) Guidelines for the early management of adults with ischemic stroke. *Stroke* **38**, 1655–711.

Bernhardt J, Dewey H, Thrift A, Collier J, Donnan G. (2008) A very early rehabilitation trial for stroke (AVERT): phase II safety and feasibility. *Stroke* **39**, 390–6.

Chiuve SE, Rexrode KM, Spiegelman D, Logroscino G, Manson JE, Rimm EB. (2008) Primary prevention of stroke by healthy lifestyle. *Circulation* **118**, 947–54.

Dempfle CE, Hennerici MG. (2011) Fibrinolytic treatment of acute ischemic stroke for patients on new oral anticoagulant drugs. *Cerebrovas Dis* **32**, 616–19.

European Stroke Organization (ESO) Executive Committee, ESO Writing Committee. (2008) Guidelines for management of ischaemic stroke and transient ischaemic attack 2008. *Cerebrovasc Dis* **25**, 457–507.

Finfer S, Chittock DR, Su SY, et al. (2009) Intensive versus conventional glucose control in critically ill patients. *N Engl J Med* **360**, 1283–97.

Hacke W, Donnan G, Fieschi C, et al. (2004) Association of outcome with early stroke treatment: pooled analysis of ATLANTIS, ECASS, and NINDS rt-PA stroke trials. *Lancet* **363**, 768–74.

Morgenstern LB, Bartholomew LK, Grotta JC, Staub L, King M, Chan W. (2003) Sustained benefit of a community and professional intervention to increase acute stroke therapy. *Arch Intern Med* **163**, 2198–202.

Wahlgren N, Ahmed N, Davalos A, et al. (2007) Thrombolysis with alteplase for acute ischaemic stroke in the Safe Implementation of Thrombolysis in Stroke-Monitoring Study (SITS-MOST): an observational study. *Lancet* **369**, 275–82.

Chapter 11

Specific treatment of acute ischaemic stroke

> **Key points**
>
> - Intravenous administration of alteplase within 3hr to onset has been the only approved specific medical therapy for the treatment of patients with acute ischaemic stroke. Recent data suggesting a benefit of therapy up to 4.5hr resulted in approval of this time window. However earlier treatment (<90min) is more likely to result in a favourable outcome.
> - In carefully selected patients interventional approaches might be an option for treatment in a stroke centre with experienced specialists.
> - In patients with BA occlusion, treatment should be initiated as soon as possible. In many stroke unit settings this means starting iv thrombolysis and considering additonal ia thrombolysis.
> - In patients <60yrs with malignant MCA stroke early hemicraniectomy reduces mortality and might improve long-term outcome.

Acute cerebral ischaemia is caused by blockage of a cerebral blood vessel, usually caused by thrombosis or embolism. Following vessel occlusion, the infarct is surrounded by an expanding area of poorly perfused tissue (the ischaemic penumbra), which is at risk for infarction, but might be salvaged if perfusion is restored within a critical time period. Therefore, specific treatment aims at reperfusion and, to be successful, reperfusion must be accomplished quickly and permanently, before the ischaemic penumbra is completely lost.

11.1 **Thrombolytic therapy**

11.1.1 **Intravenous tissue plasminogen activator**

The first small controlled trials of thrombolysis were initiated nearly 40 years ago; nowadays intravenous thrombolytic therapy is widely accepted. The National Institute of Neurological Disorders and Stroke trial (NINDS trial) showed a benefit of intravenous thrombolytic treatment (0.9mg/kg) if started within 180 min after onset of symptoms. Other studies of alteplase in acute stroke failed to demonstrate similar efficacy in a larger (0–6hr) time window for treatment (ECASS), although the risk of bleeding complications was small and a better outcome was achieved in patients with mild/moderate deficits and small infarcts on CT (ECASS II). A pooled analysis of individual data of alteplase trials showed that earlier treatment results in a better outcome, even though this analysis suggested a benefit up to 4.5hr. This was confirmed in a recently published study (ECASS III) showing that intravenous alteplase administered between 3 and 4.5hr (median 3hr 59min) after the onset of symptoms significantly improved clinical outcomes in patients with acute ischaemic stroke compared with placebo. Mortality did not differ significantly, although alteplase, increased the risk of intracerebral haemorrhage (2.4% vs 0.2%). This study reconfirmed that treatment benefit is time-dependent. The number needed to treat (NNT) to get one more favourable outcome decreased from 2 during the first 90min to 7 within 3hr, and to 14 between 3 and 4.5hr (Figure 11.1). In an observational study the SITS (Safe Implementation of Thrombolysis in Stroke) investigators compared 664 patients with ischaemic stroke treated between 3 and 4.5hr with about 10.000 patients treated within 3hr according to the official approval. There were no significant differences between the 3–4.5hr cohort and the 3-hr cohort for any outcome measures. This study confirmed in the forefront of ECASS III that alteplase remains safe in a clinical setting, when given between 3 and 4.5hr after the onset of symptoms in ischaemic stroke patients. In November 2011 the EMEA approved the application of alteplase within 4.5 hrs after onset of symptoms.

To summarize, intravenous administration of alteplase within 3–4.5hr of symptom onset is the only approved specific medical therapy for the treatment of patients with acute ischaemic stroke (Table 11.1). Earlier treatment (<90min) is more likely to result in a favourable outcome. Caution is advised before giving intravenous alteplase to people with severe stroke (NIH Stroke Scale score >25), or if CT demonstrates extended early changes of a major infarction, such as sulcal effacement, mass effect, and oedema. Treatment of patients >80 years has not been approved, but several studies demonstrated that these patients also seem to benefit despite an increased morbidity and mortality in general. However, specific risks

Fig 11.1 Relation of stroke onset to start of intravenous alteplase treatment with excellent functional outcome.

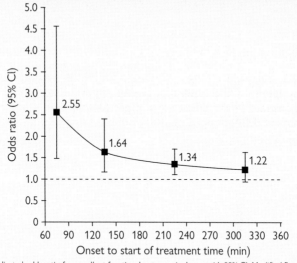

Adjusted odds ratio for excellent functional outcome is shown with 95% CI. Modified Rankin score 0–1. (From Saver, 2010).

Table 11.1 Guidelines for using alteplase to treat ischaemic stroke

Dose

- 0.9mg/kg, max. 90mg, with 10% of the dose given as a bolus followed by a 60-min infusion

Major Inclusion Criteria

- Patient >18 and <80 years; alteplase may also be administered in selected patients under 18 years and over 80 years of age, although this is outside the current European labeling (IST-3 2012)
- Treatment is recommended within 4.5 hours of onset of ischaemic stroke
- Pretreatment systolic blood pressure ≤185 mmHg and diastolic blood pressure ≤110 mmHg
- Pretreatment blood glucose concentration ≥50 mg/dL and ≤400 mg/dL
- Patient not currently taking an oral anticoagulant
- Platelet count ≥100,000/mm³

Individual therapeutic decision should be made in patients with minor neurological signs and those with major deficits. Further aspects taken into consideration include recent surgery, head trauma, major bleeding and major stroke. The patient or family members should be informed to understand the potential risks and benefits from treatment.

associated with alteplase (e.g. ICH) are not increased. Thrombolytic therapy should be given only if the diagnosis is established by a physician who has expertise in the diagnosis of stroke, and a CT or MRI scan of the brain is assessed by a physician who has expertise in reading this imaging study. Because the use of thrombolytic drugs carries the real risk of a fatal bleeding, the risks and potential benefits of alteplase should be discussed whenever possible with the patient and family before treatment is initiated. Because time is critical, thrombolytic therapy should not be delayed while waiting for the results of the prothrombin time, activated partial thromboplastin time, or platelet count unless a bleeding abnormality or thrombocytopenia is suspected, the patient has been taking warfarin and heparin, new anticoagulants (e.g. dabigatran, rivaroxaban, apixaban), or anticoagulation use is uncertain (recommendations of the American Heart Association).

An increasing number of reports have suggested that the current time window may be extended by using modern MR imaging-based selection algorithms. The underlying assumption is that the area of decreased diffusion represents the ischaemic core of the infarct and the perfusion/diffusion mismatch the critically hypoperfused, yet potentially salvageable brain tissue (ischaemic penumbra). In many dedicated stroke centres, patients with such an magnetic resonance imaging (MRI) proven perfusion-weighted MRI (PWI)/diffusion-weighted imaging (DWI) mismatch are thrombolysed even after the 4.5-hr time-window as specified by their local treatment guidelines. The multicenter WAKE UP trial tests the efficacy and safety of MRI in patients whose stroke occurred during sleep. DWI and FLAIR measurements are used to predict time from symptom onset to identify patients with acute stroke who are likely to benefit from thrombolysis. Due to strict study protocols focusing on anterior circulation stroke—mostly in the middle cerebral artery territory— there is limited data on thrombolysis in PCA stroke, but recent MRI case series have identified very comparable constellations as in anterior circulation stroke.

11.1.2 **Other intravenous thrombolytic agents**

All streptokinase trials (MAST-I, MAST-E and ASK) had to be stopped prematurely because of an excess risk of death and intracranial bleeding. In two first studies, desmoteplase—a highly fibrin-specific and non-neurotoxic thrombolytic agent—was administered intravenously 3–9h after acute ischaemic stroke in patients selected with perfusion/diffusion mismatch in MRI. Desmoteplase was associated with a higher rate of reperfusion and better clinical outcome compared with placebo. However, these findings were not confirmed in the phase III DIAS (Desmoteplase in Acute Ischemic Stroke)-II study. Ancrod, another biological thrombolytic agent also failed to show significant improvement vs. placebo despite a trend towards better clinical outcome and lack of increased ICH if administered in a 6hr window (ESTAT).

11.1.3 Intra-arterial thrombolytic therapy

After 3hr intra-arterial thrombolytic treatment is effective and safe, as shown in the Pro-urokinase in Acute Cerebral Thromboembolism II (PROACT-II) trial. Treatment with pro-urokinase started within 6 hr in patients with angiographically documented MCA occlusion led to reperfusion (66% with pro-urokinase plus heparin vs 18% with heparin alone) and a better outcome. However, conventional angiography was needed to identify eligible patients, a procedure that is not always readily available and not useful for patient selection: among 474 patients studied with angiography, only 180 were finally recruited in the study. Therefore, a very large number of patients were subjected to a small, but significant risk of increased morbidity and mortality. Since pro-urokinase is not available this treatment has been abandoned in favour of intra-arterial thrombolysis with alteplase although this has not been substantiated by randomized clinical trials (RCTs). In most stroke centres intra-arterial thrombolysis in MCA ischaemia is only performed in carefully selected patients on an individual off-label use.

11.1.4 Combined (intravenous and intra-arterial) thrombolysis

Based on pathophysiological mechanisms a combined intravenous and intra-arterial thrombolysis ('bridging technique') seems to be an opportunity to combine prompt effect (intravenous) and selectivity (intra-arterial) in the treatment of acute ischaemic stroke. This approach might be considered in particular in distal occlusion of the ICA, also termed carotid-T occlusion. Uncontrolled observational studies showed the feasibility of this approach. A randomized trial comparing standard intravenous alteplase with a combined intravenous and intra-arterial approach (The Interventional Management of Stroke, IMS3) has prematurely been stopped for futility reasons.

11.1.5 Thrombolysis in basilar artery occlusion

Despite recent advances in the treatment of acute stroke, the rate of death or disability associated with BA occlusion is almost 80%. Intra-arterial treatment of acute basilar occlusion with urokinase or alteplase has been clinically applied for more than 20 yrs, but has not been tested in an adequately powered RCT. Results from several observational studies showed no significant differences between intravenous or intra-arterial thrombolysis for BA occlusion. A recent prospective, international observational study of consecutive patients who presented with an acute symptomatic BA occlusion (n = 619) and were treated according to institutional guidelines of the participating centres (BASICS) suggested a difference in the efficacy of treatment strategies depending on the severity of the stroke. Patients with a

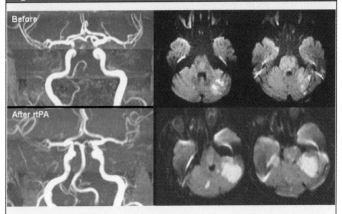

Fig 11.2 Successful treatment in BA occlusion.

Before

After rtPA

A 77 year-old woman presented with slight vertigo, dysarthria and hemihypaesthesia, onset 9.5 hours prior to admission. Symptoms were progressive up to state of coma 2.5 hours later. MRI showed an occlusion of the BA with extendend hyperacute ischaemic lesions in the brainstem and cerebellum. After intravenous alteplase treatment, MRI showed a recanalization of the BA and ischaemic lesions in both cerebellar hemispheres; however ischaemic lesions in the brainstem were clearly regressive. The mRS after 1 month was 1.

mild-to-moderate deficit more often had a poor outcome if they were treated with intra-arterial thrombolysis, rather than with intravenous thrombolysis, probably because of a delay in time until reperfusion was obtained. Conversely, patients with a severe deficit seemed to benefit from both intravenous thrombolysis and intra-arterial thrombolysis (Figure 11.2). These results should encourage clinicians to treat patients who have acute symptomatic BA occlusion with intravenous thrombolysis immediately. In case of subsequent acute worsening, additional intra-arterial thrombolysis can be considered. See Figure 11.2.

11.2 **Further developments**

11.2.1 **Intra-arterial recanalization devices**

The MERCI (Mechanical Embolus Removal in Cerebral Embolism) trial evaluated two different devices that removed the thrombus from an intracranial artery (multicentre, prospective, single-arm trial). Recanalization was achieved in 48–57.3% depending on the applied device and in 69.5% after adjunctive therapy of patients in whom the device was deployed within 8 hr of the onset of stroke symptoms. Clinically significant procedural complications occurred in 5.5% of the patients. A recently published prospective cohort study (REcanalization using Combined intravenous Alteplase and Neurointerventional ALgorithm for acute Ischaemic StrokE,

RECANALISE) showed a higher rate of recanalization in patients treated with an iv endovascular approach. New promising devices and techniques for recanalization are developed continuously. Other smaller trials testing the use of an aspiration device (Penumbra Pivotal Stroke Trial), and more recently of self-expanding stents have shown very good recanalization rates. However, whether these techniques lead to a better functional outcome remains to be shown.

11.2.2 Sonothrombolysis

Ultrasound *per se* has a thrombolytic capacity that can be used for pure mechanical thrombolysis or improvement of enzyme-mediated thrombolysis. Animal and clinical studies of sonothrombolysis have shown clot lysis, and accelerated recanalization of arterial occlusion has been seen in *in vitro* flow models. Controlled clinical trials to test safety management and effectiveness of both strategies are in progress, one randomized phase II trial (TRUMBI) showed bioeffects from low-frequency ultrasound that caused an increased rate of cerebral haemorrhage in patients concomitantly treated with intravenous alteplase. Another small randomized trial (CLOTBUST) of 2MHz transcranial ultrasound vs placebo in patients who received intravenous alteplase showed improved arterial recanalization, but failed to demonstrate any clinical benefit. A further approach is the additional administration of microbubbles, which may enhance the effect of ultrasound on thrombolysis, but also increase side effects: a first phase 2 study (TUCSON) was stopped prematurely due to safety reasons and failed to show a benefit when compared with standard intravenous alteplase therapy.

11.3 Early treatment of brain oedema and elevated intracranial pressure

Neurological deterioration due to increasing brain oedema is a common course in patients who have suffered massive stroke. Brain oedema occurs during the first hours after infarction, reaches a maximum volume at 2–4 days and is the main reason for early clinical deterioration. The effects of cerebral oedema are a further compromise of blood flow and mass effect, brain shift, and eventually potentially fatal brain herniation.

11.3.1 Medical treatment

Several treatments for post-ischaemic brain oedema are currently employed. Basic management of elevated intracranial pressure (ICP) following stroke includes positioning the patient's head at an elevation of up to 30%, avoiding noxious stimuli, pain relief, appropriate oxygenation, and normalizing body temperature. Traditionally, the mainstay of conventional therapy has consisted of ventilation, sedation, blood pressure monitoring, hyperventilation, osmotic agents, and barbiturates. If ICP monitoring is available, cerebral perfusion pressure should be kept higher than 70mmHg. The recommendations for these therapies are based upon small case series, or evidence from animal experiments. None of them has been evaluated in a randomized study. Whether ICP monitoring should be included in the routine management of patients with large strokes is still a matter of controversy.

Hypertonic, low-molecular-weight solutions such as mannitol, sorbitol, glycerol, or hypertonic saline are used to reduce the brain water content by creating an osmotic gradient between brain and plasma, drawing water into the plasma. Although strong evidence is lacking, osmotherapy with 10% glycerol, usually given intravenously (4 × 250mL of 10% glycerol over 30–60min), or intravenous mannitol (25–50g every 3–6hr) is the first medical treatment to be used if clinical and/or radiological signs of space-occupying oedema occur. The long-term effects of repeated treatments with hypertonic solutions are still unknown. Repeated infusions of mannitol 20% may aggravate cerebral oedema if the osmotic substances migrate through a damaged blood–brain barrier (BBB) into the brain tissue, reversing the osmotic gradient. Furthermore, osmotic agents predominantly lead to dehydration and shrinkage of normal brain tissue and may facilitate displacement of brain tissue and even increase the risk of herniation. However, to date, these largely theoretical considerations have not been substantiated in clinical studies.

In principle, the same dilemma applies to all other treatment strategies: They can transiently decrease elevated ICP, whereas the long-term effects are less certain or even potentially noxious. Hyperventilation induces cerebral vasoconstriction via serum and CSF alkalosis, thereby reducing the cerebral blood volume and reducing ICP. Hyperventilation can critically reduce the CBF, leading to additional ischaemic damage. Therefore, the CO_2 levels should not fall <30mmHg. Short-acting barbiturates are frequently used in patients with elevated ICP. However, their use is limited due to various side effects, such as hypotension, cardiac depression, hepatotoxicity, and predisposition to infection.

11.3.2 **Decompressive surgery**

To provide additional space for the expanding, infarcted brain tissue, extended craniectomy with dural augmentation or lobectomy has repeatedly been employed in patients with large supratentorial and cerebellar infarcts. Several authors compared decompressive surgery with conventional medical treatment and drew the conclusion that operative treatment not only reduces mortality, but may also improve functional outcome in surviving patients. If decompressive surgery is considered as a treatment option, it should probably be performed as soon as possible: most authors agree that mortality remains high in patients who already show clinical signs of tentorial herniation and brainstem compression at the time of surgery, such as loss of consciousness or pupillary abnormalities. Even in this patient group, the survival rate may be still higher than for a medically-treated patient collective. However, more disability may be expected in older patients (>55yrs of age) and in patients with dominant hemispheric infarctions (Figure 11.3). Although decompressive surgery is increasingly being used, the ideal candidate for surgery, the optimum point of time, and surgical technique are still the subject of debate. Pooled data from three controlled but small trials (VISTA, DESTINY, HALET) indicate that in patients with malignant MCA infarction, early decompressive surgery (within 48hr) may reduce mortality and increase the number of patients with a favourable functional outcome. In space-occupying cerebellar infarcts with brainstem compression it seems reasonable to consider decompressive surgery with the first signs of decreased consciousness on an individual treatment decision—no data from RCTs are available, however.

11.3.3 **Hypothermia**

Animal experiments have consistently shown that induced hypothermia (i.e. brain temperature lower than 32°C and 33°C at least) has a neuroprotective effect after focal and global ischaemia. Various mechanisms of action have been proposed, including reduced cerebral metabolism and ICP, decreased release of excitotoxic neurotransmitters, and stabilization of the BBB. However, in patients with severe, acute head trauma, who took part in a recent controlled multicentre study,

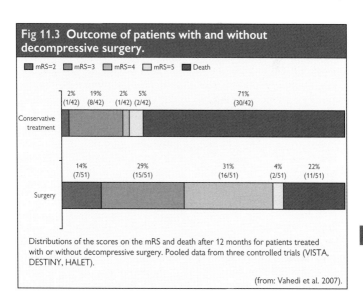

Fig 11.3 Outcome of patients with and without decompressive surgery.

■ mRS=2   ■ mRS=3   □ mRS=4   □ mRS=5   ■ Death

Conservative treatment: 2% (1/42), 19% (8/42), 2% (1/42), 5% (2/42), 71% (30/42)

Surgery: 14% (7/51), 29% (15/51), 31% (16/51), 4% (2/51), 22% (11/51)

Distributions of the scores on the mRS and death after 12 months for patients treated with or without decompressive surgery. Pooled data from three controlled trials (VISTA, DESTINY, HALET).

(from: Vahedi et al. 2007).

there wasn't any evident benefit from hypothermia. Rather in comparative trial hypothermia had more severe side effects (mainly from cardiac arrhythmia after re-warming). Indications as well as optimum temperature, duration of hypothermia, cooling and re-warming techniques, and efficacy of hypothermia are issues being addressed in larger controlled trials currently in progress (EURO Hyp).

References

Dempfle CE, Hennerici MG, . (2011) Fibrinolytic treatment of acute ischaemic stroke for patients on new oral anticoagulant drugs. *Cerebrovasc Dis* **32**, 616–19.

European Stroke Organization (ESO) Executive Committee, ESO Writing Committee. (2008) Guidelines for management of ischaemic stroke and transient ischaemic attack. *Cerebrovasc Dis* **25**, 457–507.

Hacke W, Donnan G, Fieschi C, et al. (2004) Association of outcome with early stroke treatment: pooled analysis of ATLANTIS, ECASS, and NINDS rt-PA stroke trials. *Lancet* **363**, 768–74.

Hacke W, Kaste M, Bluhmki E, et al. (2008) Thrombolysis with alteplase 3 to 4.5 hours after acute ischaemic stroke. *N Engl J Med* **359**, 1317–29.

Hacke W, Kaste M, Olsen TS, Orgogozo JM, Bogousslavsky J. (2000) European Stroke Initiative: recommendations for stroke management. Organization of stroke care. *J Neurol* **247**, 732–48.

Hennerici MG, Kay R, Bogousslavsky J, et al. (2006) Intravenous ancrod for acute ischaemic stroke in the European Stroke Treatment with Ancrod Trial: a randomised controlled trial. *Lancet* **368**, 1871–8.

IST-3 collaborative group. (2012) The benefits and harms of intravenous thrombolysis with recombinant tissue plasminogen activator within 6 h of acute ischaemic stroke (the third international stroke trial [IST-3]): a randomised controlled trial. *Lancet* **379**, 2352–63.

Morgenstern LB, Bartholomew LK, Grotta JC, Staub L, King M, Chan W. (2003) Sustained benefit of a community and professional intervention to increase acute stroke therapy. *Arch Intern Med* **163**, 2198–202.

Saver JL, Levine SR. (2010) Alteplase for ischaemic stroke—much sooner is much better. *Lancet* **375**, 1667–8.

Vahedi K, Hofmeijer J, Juettler E, et al. (2007) DECIMAL, DESTINY, and HAMLET investigators. Early decompressive surgery in malignant infarction of the middle cerebral artery: a pooled analysis of three randomised controlled trials. *Lancet Neurol* **6**, 215–22.

Wahlgren N, Ahmed N, Davalos A, et al. (2007) Thrombolysis with alteplase for acute ischaemic stroke in the Safe Implementation of Thrombolysis in Stroke-Monitoring Study (SITS-MOST): an observational study. *Lancet* **369**, 275–82.

Wahlgren N, Ahmed N, Davalos A et al. (2008) Thrombolysis with alteplase 3-4.5 h after acute ischaemic stroke (SITS-ISTR): an observational study. *Lancet* **372**, 1303–9.

Chapter 12

Specific treatment of intracerebral haemorrhage

Key points

- In up to one-third of the patients with ICH the early phase is complicated by haematoma growth.
- Despite recent efforts to find effective treatment, therapeutic options are still limited and functional outcomes remain poor.
- Promising approaches in the treatment of ICH include better management of blood pressure, thrombolytic therapy for intraventricular haemorrhage, early haemostasis to prevent haematoma growth, and minimally invasive surgery for clot lysis.

In intracerebral haemorrhage (ICH) the initial haematoma causes an increase in local pressure and subsequent rupture of other vessels surrounding the haematoma. Serial computed tomography (CT) examinations have consistently shown that in the initial phase (particularly during the first hours) the size of the haematoma markedly increases in up to 38% of patients. Mortality and morbidity in ICH patients may be predicted by the ICH score with the components age, initial GCS, ICH volume, presence or absence of intraventricular haemorrhage, and supra- or infratentorial location (see Table 12.1). General outcome factors are shown in Fig. 12.1.

12.1 General approach

Blood pressure levels are elevated in most patients with acute ICH for the first few days. Based on pathophysiological considerations and retrospective studies of patients with acute ICH systolic blood pressure should be kept below 160–170mmHg. However, a rapid decline in blood pressure in acute ICH may be associated with increased mortality due to induced hypoperfusion with the risk

Table 12.1 Intracranial haemorrhage score: The ICH score is one of the best validated scales for predicting mortality and morbidity in ICH caused by hypertension

Component	ICH score points
GCS score	
• 3–4	2
• 5–12	1
• 13–15	0
ICH volume, cm³	
• >30	1
• <30	0
IVH	
• Yes	1
• No	0
Infratentorial origin of ICH	
• Yes	1
• No	0
Age	
• >80	1
• <80	0
Total ICH score	0–6

of secondary ischaemia. The question of which antihypertensive drug should be chosen has not been addressed in systematic studies to date. Vasodilatory drugs, such as calcium antagonists, should be avoided because of the danger of cerebral vasodilatation with increased brain oedema. In Europe, the alpha-blocker urapidil is frequently given, whereas in North America, labetalol and nitroprusside are the antihypertensive drugs of choice in many institutions. The association of high blood pressure and haematoma expansion is controversial. A recent prospective randomized controlled study—Intensive Blood Pressure Reduction in Acute Cerebral Haemorrhage Trial (INTERACT)—has not demonstrated changes in clinical outcomes with intensive blood pressure lowering; a second study is ongoing (INTERACT2), which aims to lower blood pressure ≤140 mmHg within 1 hr vs 180 mmHg in a conservative treatment strategy.

About 20% of all patients with acute ICH develop seizures within the first days of treatment. Because of the high recurrence rate, antiepileptic treatment should be started immediately. Patients who have a seizure more than 2 weeks after the onset of an intracerebral

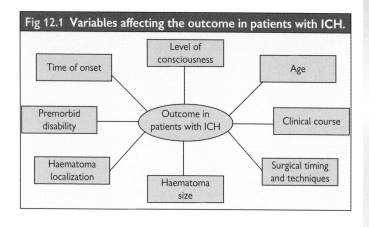

Fig 12.1 Variables affecting the outcome in patients with ICH.

Level of consciousness

Time of onset

Age

Premorbid disability

Outcome in patients with ICH

Clinical course

Haematoma localization

Haematoma size

Surgical timing and techniques

haemorrhage are at higher risk of further seizures and may require long-term prophylactic treatment with anticonvulsants. Prophylactic anti-epileptic treatment is not recommended in patients with ICH.

Although controlled studies are lacking, it is strongly recommended to meticulously treat elevated blood glucose levels. However, hypoglycaemia should also be avoided to maintain the substrate supply for the critically damaged brain tissues. Fever is an independent predictor of a poor outcome and should be rigorously treated.

Patients with ICH have an increased risk of deep vein thrombosis and pulmonary embolism. The risk and benefits of prophylactic treatment with low-dose heparin has not been sufficiently evaluated in patients with ICH. Many clinicians advocate starting prophylactic low-dose heparin therapy 24hr after the haemorrhage. Other prophylactic measures, such as compression stockings or pneumatic systems, frequent physical therapy and early mobilization may have some benefit. There is no evidence that immobilization reduces the risk of rebleeding and patients should therefore be mobilized as soon as possible.

12.2 Perifocal oedema and elevated intracranial pressure

Neurological deterioration due to increasing brain oedema is a common phenomenon in patients who have suffered an ICH. Several treatments are currently employed, in addition to general management, including positioning the head at an elevation of less than 30° and avoiding noxious stimuli. These recommendations are based on small case series, evidence from animal experiments or theoretical observations. None have been evaluated in a randomized study. In patients who need external ventricular drainage, intracranial pressure (ICP) monitoring can easily be performed. Invasive ICP monitoring is recommended infrequently, but may be beneficial in patients with a large ICH and a massive perifocal oedema to guide oedema reducing treatment.

Hypertonic solutions may be beneficial in emergency situations in an acutely deteriorating patient before therapy, such as haematoma evacuation. However, there is not enough evidence to routinely advocate osmotherapy for patients with ICH. No single therapeutic measure is of proven benefit for patients with ICH. Previously, corticosteroids were frequently employed, but after negative results from randomized studies these drugs are no longer justified. In fact, in one study the prognosis was worse in the verum group, probably due to infectious complications and hyperglycaemia.

12.3 **Specific aspects of therapy**

12.3.1 **Early progression of ICH: haemostatic treatment**

It has been proposed that early haemostatic therapy might avoid haematoma growth and, therefore improve outcome. One candidate agent was recombinant activated factor VIIa, which causes local haemostasis at sites of vascular injury by inducing local platelet aggregation when binding to the exposed subendothelial tissue factor. In a phase II trial (NovoSeven Intracerebral Haemorrhage Trial) recombinant factor VIIa successfully prevented early progression of intracerebral bleeds if administered within 3hr of onset of symptoms and suggested improved clinical outcome. However, in the phase III trial [Factor Seven for Acute Hemorrhagic Stroke (FAST)] haemostatic therapy with recombinant activated factor VII similarly reduced growth of the haematoma but failed to confirm any net benefit in survival or functional outcome.

12.3.2 **External ventricular drainage**

External ventricular drainage (EVD) is necessary in all patients with hydrocephalus. Usually, the EVD is inserted into the lateral ventricle via a frontal burr hole. In patients with massive intraventricular haemorrhage or blockage of the foramen of Monroi, the reported mortality ranges between 50% to 80%. Thus drainage of both lateral ventricles may become necessary. The EVD system is usually kept at a height of 15cm above the level of the foramen of Monroi to avoid overdrainage. If the height of the drainage system is lowered, the counterpressure subsequently decreases and a suction effect develops, which may increase the risk of rebleeding. If the hydrocephalus persists, a permanent ventriculoperitoneal shunt should be inserted as soon as the protein content of the CSF makes this intervention possible.

Intraventricular haemorrhage (IVH) commonly results from extension of ICH into the cerebral ventricular system, and is an independent predictor of mortality after ICH. Recently, intraventricular fibrinolysis with alteplase or urokinase has been repeatedly employed as an experimental therapy to speed up lysis of the intraventricular blood clot. The ongoing Phase III Clear IVH Trial (Clot Lysis Evaluating Accelerated Resolution of Intra Ventricular Haemorrhage) is designed to investigate the optimum dose and frequency of alteplase administered via an EVD to safely and effectively treat IVH.

12.3.3 Haematoma evacuation

The conventional haematoma evacuation is carried out via a small osteoplastic trepanation. A large osteoclastic trepanation may be performed only in patients who exhibit signs of tentorial herniation before surgery. Through a small cortical incision, the haematoma is removed using careful suction and irrigation. If a tumour or CAA is suspected, a biopsy should be taken for histological analysis. In the case of an angioma, a complete extirpation should be considered. Patients with CAA generally have a high rate of rebleeding, but the risk of intra- and peri-operative bleeding complications is probably not increased in this patient group.

The indications for haematoma evacuation in patients with supratentorial ICH are still unclear, and are the subject of a controversial debate. A few subsequent smaller randomized trials and several uncontrolled studies yielded inconclusive results or were negative. Most clinicians agree that comatose patients do not benefit from haematoma evacuation. Some studies have suggested that haematoma evacuation stops progressive deterioration, rather than improves overall clinical outcome. Until the benefit from haematoma evacuation is proven, the decision not to operate at all is certainly justified. A recently completed randomized controlled trial with about 1000 patients (the Surgical Trial in Intracerebral Haemorrhage [STICH]) failed to show a significant benefit of additional surgery versus medical treatment alone, however it suggested a better outcome among patients with superficial lobar haemorrhage, if treated surgically. Until generally accepted criteria are available, the indications for surgery should be established on an individual basis.

In most patients with pontine or medullar haemorrhages, a surgical haematoma evacuation is technically not possible. Although there are no data from controlled studies or guidelines, opinion-based case reports suggest that selected patients with large cerebellar ICH may benefit from haematoma evacuation. Indications for surgery in cerebellar haemorrhages are:

- A haematoma larger than 3cm in diameter
- Emergency signs of brainstem compression, such as acute loss of consciousness, abnormal pupillary responses, or pyramidal tract signs.

However, patients with cerebellar haemorrhage who present deeply comatose or with bilateral absent pupillary reflexes do not benefit from surgery. In patients with cerebellar haemorrhage, an EVD frequently becomes necessary due to obstruction of the IV ventricle from direct mechanical compression or intraventricular haemorrhage. Intracerebral bleedings from cavernomas may only be considered for surgery in case of repeat bleedings, if located in easily accessible regions or if sources of intractable seizures.

12.3.4 Treatment of arteriovenous malformations

Treatment options of AVMs are surgical resection, endovascular treatment, and radiotherapy. While the best-known therapy is surgical resection, embolization to reduce the vasculature, and radiotherapy are being used increasingly. There is a controversy whether or not AVMs that have not bled should be treated because of the possible fatal complications of therapy. The benefit of intervention for these patients is being studied by means of an international trial (ARUBA).

References

Mayer SA, Brun NC, Begtrup K, et al. (2008) Efficacy and safety of recombinant activated factor VII for acute intracerebral hemorrhage. *N Engl J Med* **358**, 2127–37.

Mendelow AD, Gregson BA, Fernandes HM, et al. (2005) Early surgery versus initial conservative treatment in patients with spontaneous supratentorial intracerebral haematomas in the International Surgical Trial in Intracerebral Haemorrhage (STICH): A randomised trial. *Lancet* **365**, 387–97.

Mohr JP, Moskowitz AJ, Stapf C, et al. (2010) The ARUBA trial: current status, future hopes. *Stroke* **41**, 537–40.

Nyquist P. (2010) Management of acute intracranial and intraventricular haemorrhage. *Crit Care Med* **38**, 946–53.

Rincon F, Mayer SA. (2010) Intracerebral haemorrhage: getting ready for effective treatments. *Curr Opin Neurol* **23**, 59–64.

Steiner T, Bösel J. (2010) Options to restrict hematoma expansion after spontaneous intracerebral haemorrhage. *Stroke.* **41**, 402–9.

Chapter 13

Specific treatment of subarachnoid haemorrhage and cerebral venous thrombosis

Key points

- Subarachnoid haemorrhage (SAH) due to rupture of an intracranial aneurysm is associated with a high risk of rebleeding and other complications, therefore early intensive care management is indicated.
- Microsurgical clipping and endovascular coiling are available for early treatment of aneurysmal SAH and are both safe and effective. If feasible, endovascular treatment is associated with a lower long-term mortality.
- Unruptured intracranial aneurysms may require preventive treatment regimens, depending on patient age, size, and site of the aneurysm.
- Intravenous or subcutaneous heparin may be considered for treatment of cerebral venous thrombosis with severe clinical presentation, although scientific evidence is lacking.

13.1 Subarachnoid haemorrhage

Subarachnoid haemorrhage (SAH) is most often due to rupture of intracranial aneurysms. Less frequently non-aneurysm bleedings from small vessels and capillaries present as perimesencephalic SAH. Intracranial aneurysms are present in about 5% of the population, most are asymptomatic and never detected. They develop during childhood/adulthood typically. Growth and formation are associated with age, hypertension, pre-existing family conditions and smoking. Treatment methods include two specific interventional options: clipping of the aneurysm and endovascular coiling (with stent-assisted coiling or flow diversion stents). Both methods are safe and effective alternative treatments and individual treatment choices should consider such parameters as aneurysm size, location, patient medical history, and operator experience. This decision should best be made in centers where both options can be offered with similarly good expertise.

13.1.1 **General management and prognosis**

In subarachnoid haemorrhage (SAH), careful monitoring and management of blood pressure is particularly important. Hypertension must be avoided because it may carry the risk of early rebleeding. However, episodes of abrupt hypotension may be associated with a worse outcome. The aim of blood pressure management is to achieve systolic values within the range 130–160mmHg. Pain should be adequately treated, and many patients will need intravenous opioids. In agitated patients, sedation is necessary. Short-acting or reversible sedatives are preferable so as not to mask clinical worsening due to hydrocephalus or rebleeding. The efficacy of corticosteroids is not established. Seizures are frequent and should be treated immediately; prophylactic anti-epileptic treatment is not recommended.

Intubation and mechanical ventilation may be indicated in patients with severe clinical deficits. Medical complications of SAH during the acute phase include neurogenic pulmonary oedema, cardiac arrhythmia, hyponatraemia, and volume depletion, presumably due to an inappropriate release of antidiuretic hormone. These complications are frequent and may require immediate symptomatic treatment.

Rebleeding after SAH is a strong predictor of a poor outcome, which occurs in about a quarter of all patients during the first 2 weeks after the first haemorrhage. The mortality from rebleeding is approximately 70%. The risk for rebleeding is greatest during the first two days after presentation. Acute worsening of neurological symptoms, sudden loss of consciousness or an otherwise unexplained increase in blood pressure should raise the suspicion of rebleeding.

Given its benign prognosis, the recommended approach for treating *perimesencephalic SAH* comprises symptomatic care with monitoring of vital parameters and careful clinical follow-up after angiographic exclusion of treatable bleeding sources.

13.1.2 **Surgical treatment of aneurysmal SAH**

Microsurgical preparation and clipping of the aneurysm is an effective and safe method to prevent further bleeding in patients with a favourable clinical status (Figure 13.1). The surgical complications and morbidity depend on several factors such as size, morphology and location of the aneurysm, presence of brain oedema or intracerebral haematoma, and the neurological status.

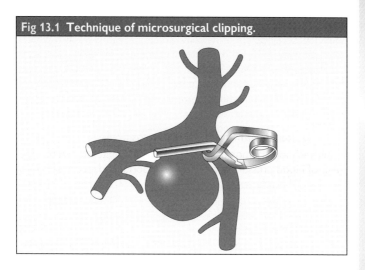

Fig 13.1 Technique of microsurgical clipping.

Most clinicians recommend operating within the first days after SAH before vasospasms have developed. Early aneurysm operation is especially indicated for patients who are alert, have little or no neurological deficit (a Hunt and Hess clinical grade of 1, 2, or 3), have no CT evidence of brain swelling, have an aneurysm that can be clipped without excessive retraction, and are considered to be clinically stable. The complication rate of surgery is markedly increased if vasospasms are already present. Another reason for an early operation is that medical treatment for vasospasm, such as induced hypertension, hypervolaemia and haemodilution ('triple-H therapy'), are feasible only if the aneurysm is safely occluded. It is seen as controversial whether patients with SAH and a severe neurological deficit (Hunt and Hess clinical grade IV and V) benefit from early surgery given the high peri-operative mortality (15–30%) and poor overall prognosis (80–90% mortality rate within the first 30 days). In these patients, supportive treatment is generally preferable. If the patients improve with supportive treatment, more aggressive diagnostic and therapeutic procedures can be pursued.

Up to 40% of patients with SAH suffer from a concomitant intracerebral haematoma, which may need immediate evacuation or ventriculostomy. In most patients, an EVD or lumbar catheter needs to be inserted because of hydrocephalus. About half of these patients require a permanent shunt at a later date.

For many years, removal of the subarachnoid blood has been advocated to reduce the severity of vasospasm and delayed ischaemic deficits. To date, the evidence supporting aggressive surgical techniques to remove the subarachnoid blood clot or instillation of fibrinolytic agents is not strong enough to recommend either as standard therapy.

13.1.3 **Endovascular treatment of intracranial aneurysms**

Since the development of flexible, directional catheters with detachable platinum coils, endovascular treatment is increasingly used to treat aneurysmal SAH (Figure 13.2). With this method, platinum coils can be inserted into the aneurysm and induce thrombosis of the lumen. The intervention is performed under general anaesthesia. Potential complications include rupture of the aneurysmal sac, incomplete occlusion, and distal embolization. Endovascular treatment seems advantageous in particular in patients with an aneurysm of the posterior circulation, where surgery carries an increased risk of operative morbidity. However, when the aneurysm is located in more distal arteries (e.g. at the trifurcation of the MCA) or involves arterial branches originating in the aneurysmal sac, or when the aneurysm has a broad base, endovascular treatment may not be possible.

The International Subarachnoid Aneurysm Trial (ISAT) was a randomized controlled trials (RCT) comparing endovascular treatment with conventional aneurysm surgery in 2143 patients with ruptured intracranial aneurysms (Figure 13.3); long-term results of this trial were published in 2009. The risk of death at 5yrs was significantly

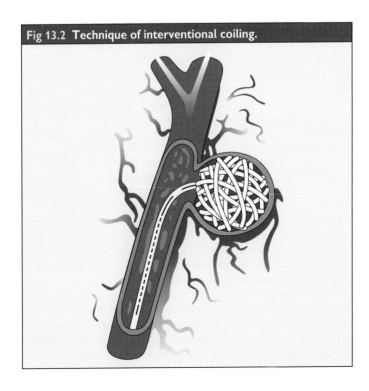

Fig 13.2 Technique of interventional coiling.

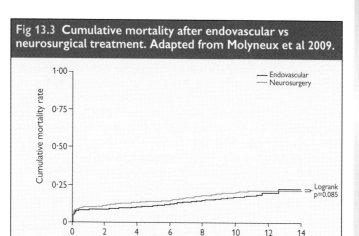

Fig 13.3 Cumulative mortality after endovascular vs neurosurgical treatment. Adapted from Molyneux et al 2009.

Endovascular	1073	(88)	979	(16)	949	(21)	905	(25)	580	(10)	266	(4)	55	(1)	0
Neurosurgery	1070	(115)	949	(22)	913	(15)	875	(30)	565	(9)	244	(3)	56	(0)	0

Number at risk (deaths)

lower in the coiling group (11%) than in the clipping group (14%), but there were no difference in rate of disability among survivors (83% vs. 82%). The risk for late rebleeding is higher after endovascular treatment, but overall rebleeding rates were low with both techniques. In summary, current data suggest that both methods are safe and effective, although endovascular treatment, when technically feasible, carries a smaller risk of early complications associated with a lower perioperative mortality, but carries a small but higher risk of recurrent bleeding, most of which are related to the treated aneurysm. Early benefits thus seemed to be lost with long-term follow-up. However, in both groups treated in ISAT, rebleeding occurred in patients with untreated and de novo aneurysms, which confirms previous observations suggesting a >20 fold greater risk of SAH in these patients. This underlines the need to better manage patients' risk factors responsible for growth and formation of new aneurysms in particular if hereditary aspects are known.

13.1.4 Management of vasospasms

Vasospasm is one of the major complications following SAH—often suspected to cause delayed cerebral ischaemia, which may be a too simplistic explanation of a complex process itself. One-third of all patients suffer from symptomatic delayed cerebral ischaemia. Without treatment, the outcome of delayed cerebral ischaemia is poor, resulting in death in roughly one-third and permanent disability in a further third of the affected patients. Current explanations blame the amount of arterial subarachnoid blood irrespective of its distribution and the degree of clinical deterioration——but possibly due to early global ischaemia as an independent predictor for poor outcome (van Gijn et al. 2007).

There is no uniformly accepted therapy for cerebral vasospasm. Triple-H therapy (arterial hypertension, hypervolaemia, haemodilution) was first advocated in 1973 and is still the conventional treatment. Triple-H therapy is started after the onset of neurological symptoms due to vasospasms. The target is a mean arterial blood pressure of 90–100mmHg after the occlusion of the aneurysm.

Many patients with SAH have spontaneously elevated blood pressure, and induced hypertension is often not necessary to reach the target mean arterial blood pressure. Volume expansion is accomplished by infusion of colloid fluids. Under this therapy, a 20% rise of the mean arterial blood pressure and a 10% decrease of the haematocrit level should be achieved. This treatment can be maintained for 10–14 days, depending on the course of the vasospasm. It is important to note that although triple-H therapy is generally accepted to be useful, this has not been unequivocally demonstrated by a prospective controlled trial. However, because of the abundant experience from uncontrolled trials, triple-H therapy can be recommended for treating vasospasm after SAH if there are no contraindications (e.g. pulmonary oedema or heart failure). In patients with untreated aneurysm, triple-H therapy may be harmful because an increased blood flow and pressure may predispose to rebleeding. Prophylactic triple-H therapy in cases without evidence of vasospasms has recently been shown not to be efficacious and should not be given.

Prophylactic administration of calcium antagonists and in particular oral nimodipine (60mg every 4hr for the first 21 days) has shown to reduce the proportion of patients with poor outcome after SAH (RRR 18%, ARR 5.1% according to a Cochrane review), although an effect on the case fatality rate has not been clearly demonstrated. The mechanism of action of nimodipine is uncertain. Nimodipine does not significantly reduce the degree of vasospasm, as was previously believed, but it probably has neuroprotective effects and may improve the microvascular collateral circulation. Because of the hypotensive effects of nimodipine, the dose may need to be reduced or a vasopressor agent given in addition. Minor side effects include flush, headache, tachycardia, and peripheral oedema.

13.1.5 **Management of unruptured aneurysms**

Unruptured cerebral aneurysms may be diagnosed in patients with SAH at the time of rupture of another aneurysm, as an incidental finding or in an elective examination (e.g. if relatives are known to have suffered from SAH). Decision-making in these patients is difficult because the risks of bleeding and of potential complications from therapeutic interventions need to be well known and balanced. According to

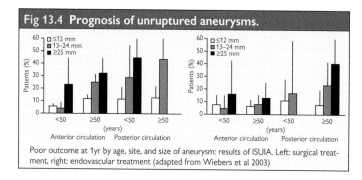

Fig 13.4 Prognosis of unruptured aneurysms.

Poor outcome at 1yr by age, site, and size of aneurysm: results of ISUIA. Left: surgical treatment, right: endovascular treatment (adapted from Wiebers et al 2003)

the International Study of Unruptured Intracranial Aneurysms (ISUIA), the risk of recurrent SAH in patients with a history of SAH is high (0.5–2.4% per year). Except the aneurysm is very small or difficult to treat, intervention may be offered because these patients are not healthy but carriers of a life-threatening condition. However, in patients without prior history of ruptured aneurysm, the 5-yr cumulative rupture rates are lower and depend on various factors (Figure 13.4). Preventive treatment of non-ruptured aneurysms is recommended with aneurysms larger than 7mm, symptomatic aneurysms, and known additional risk factors. Other features that increase the risk of rupture include aneurysm formation, aneurysm growth, symptomatic aneurysms, and genetic and familial predisposition.

13.2 Cerebral venous thrombosis

13.2.1 Medical treatment of acute cerebral venous thrombosis

Since 1941, heparin has been advocated as therapy of choice for CVT. Two small placebo-controlled, randomized studies on the use of heparin yielded inconclusive results. In one study, an apparent benefit from intravenous heparin therapy was suggested despite premature stop after recruitment of 20 patients only. This study has been repeatedly criticized for several methodological problems. Another controlled trial found no significant benefit from low molecular weight heparin. In both studies, and in several uncontrolled case series, the risk of haemorrhage was not increased with heparin therapy, even in patients presenting with secondary haemorrhage. Based on these data, most experts recommend using either intravenous or subcutaneous heparin in patients with CVT, especially in those with severe clinical presentation. However, the scientific evidence supporting this practice is rather weak.

13.2.2 **Interventional therapy**

Systemic treatment with fibrinolytic agents or local fibrinolysis via a transvenous catheter with urokinase or alteplase has been repeatedly employed to hasten the recanalization of the occluded sinuses. Most case report authors describe a higher recanalization rate compared with the spontaneous course and a favourable clinical outcome after fibrinolysis; the rate of haemorrhagic complications seemed to be low; up to now, systematic studies on fibrinolytic therapy in CVT have not been performed.

13.2.3 **Secondary prophylaxis following CVT**

As with the management of patients with deep venous thrombosis of the lower limbs, oral anticoagulation with warfarin is often recommended for 3–6 months after CVT, if no indication for continuous anticoagulation is present. There are, however, no data from systematic studies supporting this strategy. In patients with CVT secondary to hypercoagulation syndromes, the underlying coagulation disorder needs to be treated. Therefore, life-long oral anticoagulation may be necessary in some patients.

References

Bousser MG. (2000) Cerebral venous thrombosis: diagnosis and management. *J Neurol* **247**, 252–8.

Currie S, Mankad K, Goddard A. (2011) Endovascular treatment of intracranial aneurysms: review of current practice. *Postgrad Med J* **87**, 41–50.

van Gijn J, Kerr RS, Rinkel GJ. (2007) Subarachnoid haemorrhage. *Lancet* **369**, 306–18.

Molyneux AJ, Kerr RS, Birks J, et al. (2009) ISAT Collaborators. Risk of recurrent subarachnoid haemorrhage, death, or dependence and standardised mortality ratios after clipping or coiling of an intracranial aneurysm in the International Subarachnoid Aneurysm Trial (ISAT): long-term follow-up. *Lancet Neurol* **8**, 427–33.

Molyneux AJ, Kerr RS, Yu LM, et al. (2005) International Subarachnoid Aneurysm Trial (ISAT) Collaborative Group. International subarachnoid aneurysm trial (ISAT) of neurosurgical clipping versus endovascular coiling in 2143 patients with ruptured intracranial aneurysms: a randomised comparison of effects on survival, dependency, seizures, rebleeding, subgroups, and aneurysm occlusion. *Lancet* **366**, 809–17.

Seibert B, Tummala RP, Chow R, et al. (2011) Intracranial aneurysms: review of current treatment options and outcomes. *Front Neurol* **2**, 45.

Sen J, Belli A, Albon H, Morgan L, Petzold A, Kitchen N. (2003) Triple-H therapy in the management of aneurysmal subarachnoid haemorrhage. *Lancet Neurol* **2**, 614–21.

Wiebers DO, Whisnant JP, Huston J 3rd, et al. (2003) International Study of Unruptured Intracranial Aneurysms Investigators. Unruptured intracranial aneurysms: natural history, clinical outcome, and risks of surgical and endovascular treatment. *Lancet* **362**, 103–10.

Secondary prevention, recovery and rehabilitation

Chapter 14

Secondary prevention

Key points

- Blood pressure lowering is recommended after the acute phase of stroke or TIA, including patients with normal blood pressure.
- Statin therapy is recommended in all patients with focal cerebral ischaemia.
- It is recommended that patients receive antiplatelet drugs (aspirin 50–100mg, clopidogrel 75mg, or aspirin 2 × 25mg plus dipyridamole 2 × 200 mg).
- Oral anticoagulation is recommended after ischaemic stroke or TIA associated with atrial fibrillation.
- Carotid endarterectomy is recommended for patients with 70–95% stenosis within few weeks after the index ischaemic event.

After a patient has had a stroke or transient ischaemic attack (TIA) there are several strategies for preventing a recurrence. These strategies depend on the mechanism of the stroke or TIA. Controlling risk factors is very important and the studies discussed for primary prevention also apply to recurrent stroke prevention, although the number of trials available supporting this hypothesis are fewer than for primary prevention. Many details discussed more extensively in Chapter 2 should be considered for secondary prevention as well (Tables 14.1, 14.2, and 4.1).

Table 14.1 Different steps in stroke prevention after TIA or first stroke (modified from Diener et al. 2010)

Type of intervention	Level of recommendation	Relative RR	Absolute RR per year	NNT per year	Remarks
Antihypertensive therapy	A	24%	0.46%	217	Well documented for perindopril, indapamide and eprosartan
Statins (Atorvastatin 80mg)	A	16%	0.4%	250	Until now documented for atorvastatin and simvastatin
ASA50-150mg	A	18–22%	1.3%	77	ASA doses >150mg = higher bleeding risk
ASA 50mg + dipyridamole	A	23%	1.0–1.5%	33–100	Combination also significantly more effective than placebo
Clopidogrel vs ASA	B	8%	0.5%	200	Based on a subgroup analysis of the CAPRIE-study
Carotid surgery Carotid stenting	A	65%	3.1%	32	Surgery more effective and less risks than carotid stenting
Oral anticoagulation (warfarin) in aimed INR = 2.0–3.0	A	68%	8%	12	New anticoagulants (e.g. dabigatran, rivaroxaban etc.) show less risk of severe bleeding events and better prevention of ischaemia
ASA in AF	A	19%	2.5%	40	Better than placebo, but inferior to apixaba

*Endpoint stroke and death; NNT = number needed to treat; RR = risk reduction; AF = atrial fibrillation.

Table 14.2 Model for risk evaluation of a recurrence insult after a first ischaemic event, based on the Essen Risk Score. A score of ≥3 points means a recurrent stroke risk of ≥4% per year (modified from Diener et al. 2010)

Risk factor	Points
<65yrs	0
65–75yrs	1
> 75yrs	2
Arterial hypertension	1
Diabetes mellitus	1
Myocardial infarction	1
Other cardiovascular events	1
Peripheral artery disease	1
Smoking	1
Additional TIA/stroke	1

14.1 **Optimal management of vascular risk factors**

14.1.1 **High blood pressure**

Hypertension is by far the most important risk factor, both for first-ever stroke and stroke recurrence. However, the only study available that showed a significant reduction in stroke recurrence with blood-pressure lowering in patients with hypertension (and what is probably more interesting, in those without hypertension, too) after a TIA or stroke, is the Perindopril pROtection aGainst REcurrent Stroke Study (PROGRESS). In this study, patients receiving a diuretic (indapamide) and an ACE inhibitor (perindopril) had a relative risk reduction of 42% for stroke, compared with placebo. Patients treated with perindopril alone did not have a lower risk of stroke than patients receiving placebo. The combination regimen also lowered blood pressure significantly more than single therapy (12/5mmHg vs 9/4mmHg), suggesting that the benefits were driven by the degree of blood pressure reduction (RR <140/90 mmHg).

The ESO recommends ACE inhibitors and diuretics for stroke prevention not only in hypertensive patients, but also in those who are normotensive, but who have additional risk factors. In both groups of patients, this recommendation is supported by data from the HOPE and LIFE primary prevention studies. Which anti-hypertensive class is the most effective in secondary prevention of stroke or TIAs is still a matter of discussion. Perindopril plus indapamide is significantly more effective than nitrendipine. Early secondary prevention with telmisartan in addition to a common antihypertensive drug showed no superiority to placebo (PROFESS). More recently, a meta-analysis by Rothwell et al. suggested that in patients after stroke or TIA the variability of blood pressure is an independent predictor of stroke (OR 6.22; CI 95% 4.16–9.29; p < 0.0001). In a subsequent analysis, the same group showed that patients treated with the calcium antagonist amlodipine had less variable blood pressure values than those treated with atenolol, which may explain the better outcome observed in the ASCOT-BLA study. Similar observations were made with diuretics, but not with ACE inhibitors or angiotensin I/II receptor antagonists (ARBs), which are particularly recommended for patients with diabetes.

14.1.2 **Diabetes mellitus**
Classical cardiovascular risk management including a 'healthy lifestyle', antihypertensive and antiplatelet drugs, as well as statins are recommended to prevent vascular complications and stroke recurrence in patients with diabetes.

Even though the rate of stroke mortality and recurrent events in type 2 diabetes is higher than in controls, sufficient prospective data on secondary stroke prevention in this population are lacking. One of the few–the prospective, double-blind PROspective pioglitAzone Clinical Trial In macroVascular Events (PROactive) study examined the effect of the thiazolidinedione pioglitazone on the risk of cardiovascular events in 5238 patients with type 2 diabetes and a history of macrovascular disease, including 984 with previous stroke. In the overall study population, pioglitazone was associated with a non-significant 19% relative risk reduction in fatal/non-fatal stroke. However, a subanalysis in patients with previous stroke showed a significant 47% relative risk reduction of recurrent strokes. Possibly due to its ability to raise high-density lipoprotein (HDL-C), the substance has also been shown to reduce the progression of atherosclerosis in patients with type 2 diabetes. However, a meta-analysis by Lincoff et al. (2007) of 19 RCTs pioglitazone vs. placebo in 16390 patients with diabetes after 4 months—3.5 years of treatment showed the expected reduction of death, myocardial infarction and stroke (HR 0.82; 0.72–0.94 and p = 0.005) but also an increased risk for serious heart failure (HR 1.41; 1.14–1.76 and p = 0.002). Whether or not pioglitazone increases insulin resistance (a potential independent risk factor for stroke) or acts in a modification of other risk factors, is an open question.

14.1.3 Hyperlipidaemia

Lipid-lowering agents have mostly been tested in patients with coronary artery disease and recent myocardial infarction, and results from subpopulations with stroke or TIA are most relevant in terms of primary prevention. However, more recent data indicate that statins are also effective in reducing stroke recurrence. A subgroup analysis of the Heart Protection Study showed a risk reduction of 4.9% in patients with a qualifying cerebrovascular event treated with 40mg simvastatin, irrespective of their initial lipid values. Due to the small number of stroke patients included in this big trial (1820 out of a total of 20,536), this result did not reach statistical significance. While PROSPER failed to show similar effects, the first analysis of the Anglo-Scandinavian Cardiac Outcome Trial Lipid Lowering Trial (ASCOT-LLT) showed—for the first time—a significant reduction in non-fatal ischaemic strokes in patients with a first TIA or stroke who were treated with atorvastatin (10mg/day) vs placebo.

In the Stroke Prevention by Aggressive Reduction in Cholesterol Levels (SPARCL) study (Amarenco et al. 2006) 4731 patients without CHD and LDL-C-levels between 100 and 190 mg/dL were treated after stroke/TIA with 80 mg atorvastatin vs. placebo. After a mean of 4.9 years fatal or non-fatal strokes (primary outcome) occurred significantly less frequent with aggressive doses of atorvastatin (11.2% vs. 13.1%, HR 0.84; 0.71–0.99 and p = 0.03). A small increase in the incidence of hemorrhagic stroke was not due to statin treatment but resulted from inclusion of 2% of patients with haemorrhagic strokes as both qualifying and recurrent events.

Sequential reports from this trial showed that patients benefitted most if a reduction of LDL-C of >50% from basal value could be achieved. Thus prevention treatment should start early after a stroke and LDL-C-levels should be controlled for dosage (target levels <100 mg/dL in secondary prevention and <70 mg/dL for people with diabetes type 2).

14.1.4 Lifestyle (cigarette smoking/obesity/physical activity)

Smoking has been identified as a risk factor for stroke and cessation has been shown to have significant effects in primary prevention. However, there is no convincing evidence that avoiding cigarette smoking after stroke plays a weighty role in secondary prevention of recurrent events. Some studies indicate that weight loss and physical exercise may be indirectly beneficial after stroke as it lowers blood pressure and reduces insulin resistance. The intake of vitamins (vitamin E, folate vitamin B6, vitamin B12) does not prevent vascular events or even may increase the risk of cardiovascular mortality (beta-carotene). Treatment of hyperhomocysteinaemia with the vitamins B6, B12, and folic acid failed to show significant effects in secondary prevention of a general stroke population; however, in patients with small vessel disease or MTHFR 677C polymorphism and specific nutritional conditions in different parts of the world, substitution seems to be beneficial (Hankey et al. 2011).

Sleep-disordered breathing represents both a risk factor and a consequence of stroke and is related to higher stroke incidence and poorer long-term outcome. Obstructive sleep apnoea is the most common cause of sleep-disordered breathing in stroke, which can be treated by continuous positive airway pressure. Physical exercise regularly performed (about twice/week) contributes to a reduction of risk factors and stroke recurrences, e.g. by reducing atherosclerotic plaque vulnerability (Szostak and Laurant 2011)

14.1.5 **Atrial fibrillation**

In patients with atrial fibrillation as a cause of first-ever stroke, oral anticoagulation with an INR of 2.0–3.0 is recommended. This evidence derives from a single study published in 1993 (EAFT) with several limitations from present perspectives. However, several meta-analyses and more robust data from primary prevention studies support the present guidelines. In cases of contraindications against anticoagulants, 300 mg aspirin is recommended if tolerated (or 100mg otherwise) but even prevention with a combination of aspirin and clopidogrel is definitely inferior to anticoagulants, and shows significant rates of severe bleeding complications. For the future apixaban might be the drug of choice in patients with AF unsuitable to vitamin K antagonists (Connolly et al. 2011). New oral antagonists (dabigatran, rivaroxaban, apixaban) may replace warfarin for a better benefit/risk ratio (see 14.2.8). In patients with other cardiogenic sources of stroke such as mechanical heart valve replacement, aneurysms after myocardial infarction, etc., anticoagulation with appropriate INR levels are strongly recommended.

There are no data available about when to start anticoagulation after the index symptoms of stroke or TIAs. Similarly no data are available about the difficult decision when anticoagulation should be restarted in patients, who had suffered from either intra- or extracerebral bleedings or after an ischaemic stroke with secondary haemorrhage or haemorrhagic transformation during such treatment. The common use of heparin treatment in an interval of 2–4 weeks lacks decent support: in contrast, it may be associated with an increased risk for bleeding complications and be less effective than anticoagulation with warfarin. Thus, heparin should only be used if substantial indications are given (e.g thrombus formation in the left atrium, ventricle or the aorta etc). Dabigatran is probably the best choice because of its pharmakokinetic characteristics.

There is no information whether or not patients with co-existing sources of stroke may benefit from long-term combined medication with anticoagulants plus antiplatelet agents (e.g. in patients with AF and significant small vessel disease, both responsible for stroke recurrences in the individual patient). Several clinical trials, testing this hypothesis, had to be stopped prematurely for safety reasons due to increased bleeding complications—thus despite potential benefits this combination should be avoided. There are, however, some situations, where this treatment (e.g. triple therapy 'TT' with aspirin, clopidogrel and anticoagulants) are needed: in patients with AF on anticoagulants, who suffer myocardial infarction and need stenting therapy. In this condition, the selection of stents is important to limit TT to a period as short as possible. In addition, clopidogrel should be replaced by prasugrel in patients with P2Y12 receptor deficiency, who do not respond to clopidogrel (~20%). New anticoagulants may hopefully provide better perspectives for this increasing group of patients as age of our populations is increasing along with both atherosclerosis and AF.

Non-pharmacological methods for managing abnormal heart rhythm exist and research is ongoing in this area, too. These include electric cardioversion, radiofrequency or kryo-ablation and interventional left atrial appendage closure. All these procedures have not been investigated with regard to their capacities in replacing anticoagulants after successful restoration of sinus rhythm (Furlan et al. 2012). Surgical procedures are being developed to reduce the risk of thrombo-embolic events reaching the brain (see Chapter 2.7).

14.1.6 Patent foramen ovale

Several case studies suggest an association between the presence of a patent foramen ovale (PFO) and cryptogenic stroke in both younger and older stroke patients. In patients with PFO combined with an atrial septal aneurysm, an Eustachian valve, a Chiari network, or in patients who have suffered more than one stroke the risk of recurrence was considered to be substantial. However, several RCTs showed that the risk is small (1–2% annually or less) and cannot be significantly reduced by medical (ASS or anticoagulation) or interventional (PFO closure) treatment. Data from the CLOSURE trial showed that a potential benefit in stroke reduction was counterbalanced by an unexpected increase in secondary complications after PFO closure (induced AF in particular) (Furlan et al. 2012).

14.2 Antithrombotic therapy

14.2.1 Antiplatelet therapy

Three antiplatelet drugs aspirin, clopidogrel and dipyridamole have been shown to be efficacious in the secondary prevention of stroke.

14.2.2 **Aspirin**

Numerous clinical trials have compared aspirin with placebo for the prevention of stroke and death after TIA or minor stroke. The Antithrombotic Trialists' Collaboration meta-analysis of 21 trials of people with a past history of stroke or TIA, reported an odds reduction of 22% for non-fatal stroke, non-fatal myocardial infarction, or vascular death with a 2-year risk of 17.8% for those treated with antiplatelets and 21.4% for controls. Similar reductions were found for women and men, young and old, hypertensives and normotensives, diabetics and non-diabetics. Recommendations for dose of aspirin ranged from 30mg/day to 1300mg/day, however, in a large meta-analysis aspirin ≥75mg was equivalent to <75mg in preventing vascular events. The risk of extracranial bleeding was similar with aspirin doses less than 325mg but considerably increased with dosage >325mg. Current recommendations are to treat stroke and TIA survivors with 50–325mg aspirin/day.

14.2.3 **Dipyridamole/Cilostazol**

Older studies have reported conflicting results about the benefit of dipyridamole for prevention of recurrent stroke as aspirin. Results from two European stroke prevention studies showed that 200mg of extended-release dipyridamole bid was as effective as 25mg aspirin bid, with the combination of the two being even better than aspirin alone for the prevention of stroke after TIA or minor stroke. The relative risk reduction of stroke or death was 13% for aspirin, 15% for dipyridamole and 24% for the combination of the two. However, the PRoFESS trial failed to show that treatment with combined aspirin/extended-release dipyridamole is superior to clopidogrel regarding functional outcome, stroke recurrence, death, bleeding, or serious adverse events. The antiplatelet drug cilostazol was studied in Asia (Chinese and Japanese populations) and significantly reduced recurrent strokes; however this was mainly due to a reduction of secondary brain haemorrhage being far more often in Asians than in Caucasians/Blacks.

14.2.4 **Clopidogrel**

The antiplatelet agent clopidogrel was studied in the Clopidogrel vs Aspirin in Patients at Risk of Ischaemic Events (CAPRIE) trial. In this study, 19,185 patients with ischaemic stroke, myocardial infarction, or peripheral vascular disease were randomized to clopidogrel 75mg vs aspirin 325mg. For the primary end point of combined stroke, myocardial infarction or vascular death, there was a relative risk reduction of 8.7% and an absolute risk reduction of 0.9% with clopidogrel over aspirin. Among the stroke subgroup, there was a 7.3% relative risk reduction of stroke, myocardial infarction, or vascular death.

14.2.5 Combination regimens

The Management of Atherothrombosis with Clopidogrel in High-risk patients with recent TIA or stroke (MATCH) trial randomized high-risk patients (prior ischaemic stroke, myocardial infarction, peripheral vascular disease or diabetes) to therapy with clopidogrel or clopidogrel plus aspirin. The trialists assessed for the outcomes of ischaemic stroke, myocardial infarction, or death at 18 months. There was no significant difference in outcome for the two treatment groups, but the combination of clopidogrel and aspirin significantly increased the risk of major bleeding events. Similarly, in the Clopidogrel for High Atherothrombotic Risk and Ischaemic Stabilization, Management and Avoidance (CHARISMA) study, the combination of aspirin and clopidogrel did not reduce the risk of stroke or death from cardiovascular causes, compared with aspirin alone.

14.2.6 Recurrent vascular events under antiplatelet therapy—new agents

In patients with recurrent vascular events under antiplatelet therapy alternative causes of stroke need to be sought and consistent risk-factor management is obligatory. There is no evidence to routinely change antiplatelet therapy, but in individual cases one might consider switching to another antiplatelet substance, adding another antiplatelet agent or even the use of oral anticoagulation if intermittent AF is suspected. Clopidogrel and aspirin is still used to prevent secondary thromboembolism and reocclusion after interventional vascular treatment (e.g. coronary artery stenting after MI and carotid stenting after stroke/TIA associated with artery-to-artery embolism). Treatment should be limited, however, to 3–12 months intervals to avoid bleeding complications (for clopidogrel non-responders see p. 153). A new antiplatelet agent terutroban was recently studied vs. aspirin in a large RCT including 19120 patients with previous stroke/TIA (PERFORM, Bousser et al. 2011). Although this selective thromboxane-prostaglandine receptor antagonist had anti-inflammatory and antithrombotic effects in addition to platelet inhibitory mechanism, the trial failed to show superiority vs. aspirin in the prevention of cerebral and cardiovascular ischaemic events (HR 1.02; 0.94–1.12 and $p > 0.05$). In a subgroup analysis terutroban was significantly better than aspirin in patients who had already suffered a previous stroke prior to the qualifying event. However, this might have been due to the large number of subanalysis requested and hence be considered an observation by chance rather than reflect a special group of aspirin non-responders.

14.2.7 Oral anticoagulation

Warfarin is an oral anticoagulant that has been demonstrated to be effective in the prevention of cardio-embolic stroke. Randomized clinical trials have evaluated the relative merits of warfarin or aspirin in patients with non-valvular AF. The European Atrial Fibrillation Trial (EAFT 1993) convincingly demonstrated that anticoagulation therapy reduced the risk of recurrent stroke in patients with AF and TIA or minor stroke from 12 to 4%, compared with placebo. The risk reduction of 67% was similar to that found in the other AF trials among people with no prior neurological events. Oral anticoagulants were more effective than aspirin, and aspirin was better than placebo—in patients with contraindications against oral anticoagulation—but the latter effect was marginal only. The combination of ASA and clopidogrel is inferior to anticoagulants but shows similar rates of severe bleeding complications. The EAFT, in conjunction with the other warfarin studies, provides support that warfarin with an INR of 2.0–3.0 is the therapy of choice in patients with a cardiac source and a TIA or minor stroke, provided there is no contraindication to its use. In patients with mechanical heart valve replacement INR values between 2.0–3.5 should be considered.

The Warfarin Aspirin Recurrent Stroke Study (WARSS) was designed to answer the question whether warfarin plays a role in the treatment of non-cardioembolic stroke or TIA. WARSS was a randomized, double-blind trial of warfarin with an INR of 1.4–2.8 vs aspirin 325mg in 2206 patients with non-cardio-embolic stroke. These patients were followed for 2yrs with the primary end point of stroke or death. Death or recurrent stroke occurred in 16.9% of patients. There was no difference between patients treated with warfarin or aspirin. There was also no difference in haemorrhage rates. Although warfarin with an INR of 1.4–2.8 appears to be safe, there was no additional benefit in preventing recurrent stroke compared to aspirin. In contrast, another study investigated warfarin and aspirin in symptomatic intracranial arterial stenosis (WASID 2005). In this trial warfarin was associated with significantly higher rates of adverse events and provided no benefit over aspirin. The European-Australian Stroke Prevention Trial (ESPRIT 2007) compared warfarin (INR 2.0–3.0) vs. ASS (300–325 mg) in patients with TIA/stroke and reported a reduction of stroke recurrences during warfarin treatment; however this advantage was balanced by an increased number of intracerebral bleedings.

14.2.8 **New antithrombotic agents**

New anticoagulants are under development in very advanced phases of clinical research. They offer reliable efficacy and tolerability with the benefit of simplified management and no need for frequent monitoring or dose adjustment. New antiplatelet agents to reduce thrombus formation are also in advanced stages of development (ticagrelor or prasugrel) but have different bleeding complication rates (ticagrelor >> prasugrel).

Oral direct factor Xa inhibitors are the most promising new drugs achieving effective anticoagulation by inhibiting thrombin generation, while allowing existing thrombin to continue its normal role in blood clotting. They include rivaroxaban, apixaban, and edoxaban and these were evaluated in primary and secondary prevention studies (related to stroke as reported on pages 21/22). ROCKET-AF (Patel et al. 2011) was a randomized, double-blind study to compare the efficacy and safety of 20mg rivaroxaban once daily with warfarin for the prevention of stroke in approximately 14,000 patients with AF. Rivaroxaban was non-inferior compared to warfarin for the prevention of stroke or systemic embolism and there were no overall differences between major bleeding risks. Intracranial and fatal bleeding, however, occurred less frequently in the rivaroxaban group.

Apixaban was evaluated for efficacy and safety in a randomized, double-blind phase III study (5mg twice daily) compared with warfarin for stroke prevention in patients with AF (ARISTOTLE, Granger et al. 2011). Apixaban was superior in preventing stroke and systemic embolism, caused less bleeding, and resulted in a lower mortality. In another phase III study has investigated apixaban vs aspirin in patients with AF for whom vitamin K antagonists were unsuitable (AVERROES, Connolly et al. 2011): this study was prematurely terminated because apixaban reduced the risk of stroke or systemic embolism without increaseing the risk of major bleeding or intracerebral haemorrhage. It is approved for treatment in patients with AF.

Dabigatran, a direct thrombin inhibitor, was evaluated in the RE-LY-study (Connolly et al. 2009), a randomized, controlled trial comparing the efficacy and safety of two blinded doses of dabigatran etexilade with open label warfarin for prevention of stroke and systemic embolism in patients with non-valvular AF; although originally designed as a non-inferiority trial, it turned out to show a benefit to prevent recurrent ischaemia and a reduced risk of severe bleeding complications for both doses and is approved for treatment in patients with AF.

14.3 **Surgery and angioplasty/stenting**

14.3.1 **Carotid endarterectomy (CEA)**

Carotid endarterectomy has been shown to reduce the risk of ischaemic stroke in patients with symptomatic carotid stenosis. The North American Symptomatic Carotid Endarterectomy Trial (NASCET) studied patients with TIA or minor stroke and an ipsilateral carotid stenosis of 70% or more (Figure 14.1). This study was stopped early because of the significant benefit seen in the surgical group. It found the 2-year risk of ipsilateral stroke was 9% in the surgical group and 26% in the medical group (aspirin 1300mg/day). The absolute risk reduction

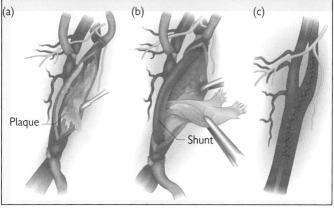

Fig 14.1 Carotid endarterectomy dissects atheromatous plaques (a) with or without shunting (b) closure can be performed directly (c) or using patch/material.

(a)   (b)   (c)

Plaque

Shunt

was 17%. Risk reductions were less for those with moderate stenosis (50–69%) and dependent on concomitant risk factors.

The Veterans Administration Cooperative Study showed that among those with greater than 50% carotid stenosis, the risk of stroke after a mean follow-up of 11.9 months was 7.7% in the surgical group and 19.4% in the non-surgical group. The European Carotid Surgery Trial (ECST) also showed a benefit for high-grade symptomatic carotid stenosis, but there was no significant benefit of surgery for those with 0–29% stenosis.

The consensus is that for patients with a TIA or minor stroke, and ipsilateral carotid stenosis of more than 70%, carotid endarterectomy is the best option for preventing a recurrent event. For those with less than 50% stenosis endarterectomy has no benefits, while for those with 50–69% stenosis and ipsilateral symptoms the use of endarterectomy depends on the risk strata of the patient. Rather than the degree of stenosis only, as evaluated by conventional angiography in the ECST and NASCET, the decision for surgery or medical treatment today follows a series of parameters to identify patients with high risk for stroke, who might benefit most from surgery (Rothwell 2004). Nowadays the degree and pattern of carotid obstructions is usually demonstrated by non-invasive methods (ultrasound and MR imaging studies).

14.3.2 **Carotid angioplasty and stenting (CAS)**

Non-surgical treatment of carotid disease with angioplasty and stent placement through endovascular techniques is becoming more widespread. It is now a technically feasible option and has initially been used in patients either because of a distal location of the stenosis or because of a high risk for undergoing anaesthesia. Studies comparing angioplasty with carotid endarterectomy have addressed issues of safety and long-term early stroke risk (Figure 14.2). In a small study, 43 patients with symptomatic carotid stenosis (≥70%) underwent stent placement. Of these, 40 patients had successful recanalization. They were followed for a mean of 20 months. Mortality at 30 days was 2.5% and the overall stroke or death rate was 5% at the end of the follow-up period.

The Wallstent study was stopped early because of worse outcome in patients who underwent stent placement over endarterectomy. The 30-day risk of stroke or death was 11 vs 5%. The Carotid and Vertebral Artery Transluminal Angioplasty Study (CAVATAS) was a larger, randomized study comparing angioplasty and endarterectomy. About 500 patients with symptomatic carotid stenosis that was deemed necessary for treatment and would be amenable to either procedure were randomized. The study found no significant difference in death or stroke between the two groups (10%). There was no difference in death, disabling stroke or non-disabling stroke. There was a lower incidence of cranial nerve palsy in the interventionally treated patients (0 vs 9%).

According to follow-up analysis in CAVATAS restenosis is about three times more common after endovascular treatment than after endarterectomy and more patients had stroke during follow-up

159

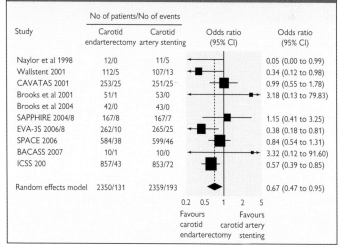

Fig 14.2 Odds ratios of risk for composite of stroke or death within 30 days of carotid endarterectomy vs carotid artery stenting.(from Meier et al. 2010)

| Study | No of patients/No of events | | Odds ratio (95% CI) | Odds ratio (95% CI) |
	Carotid endarterectomy	Carotid artery stenting		
Naylor et al 1998	12/0	11/5		0.05 (0.00 to 0.99)
Wallstent 2001	112/5	107/13		0.34 (0.12 to 0.98)
CAVATAS 2001	253/25	251/25		0.99 (0.55 to 1.78)
Brooks et al 2001	51/1	53/0		3.18 (0.13 to 79.83)
Brooks et al 2004	42/0	43/0		
SAPPHIRE 2004/8	167/8	167/7		1.15 (0.41 to 3.25)
EVA-3S 2006/8	262/10	265/25		0.38 (0.18 to 0.81)
SPACE 2006	584/38	599/46		0.84 (0.54 to 1.31)
BACASS 2007	10/1	10/0		3.32 (0.12 to 91.60)
ICSS 200	857/43	853/72		0.57 (0.39 to 0.85)
Random effects model	2350/131	2359/193		0.67 (0.47 to 0.95)

0.2 0.5 1 2 5
Favours carotid endarterectomy   Favours carotid artery stenting

in the endovascular group than in the surgical group, but the rate of ipsilateral non-peri-operative stroke was low in both groups and none of the differences in the stroke outcome measures was significant.

The SPACE study (Stent-protected Angioplasty vs Carotid Endarterectomy in symptomatic patients) failed to verify the non-inferiority of angioplasty compared to endarterectomy because numbers of patients recruited did not meet statistical significance values. The French EVA3S trial (Endarterectomy vs Stenting in Patients with Symptomatic Severe Carotid Stenosis) was stopped ahead of schedule after safety concerns and lack of efficacy, because of a higher risk of stroke and death within 30 days after angioplasty compared with endarterectomy. Results from 3433 patients with symptomatic carotid stenosis as randomly assigned and analysed in the EVA-3S, the SPACE and the ICSS trials were pooled and analysed recently (CSTC 2010). In the first 4 months after randomization any stroke or death occurred significantly more often in the CAS than in the CEA groups (HR 1.53; 1.20–1.95 and p = 0.0006). Of all subgroups investigated, only age modified the treatment effect (Figure 14.3): in patients 70 years or older, the estimated risk with CAS was twice that with CEA (HR 2.04; 1.48–2.82 and p = 0.0053).

The primary aim of the recent North American Carotid Revascularization Endarterectomy vs Stenting Trial (CREST) was to compare the outcomes of carotid-artery stenting with those of carotid endarterectomy among both patients with symptomatic and asymptomatic

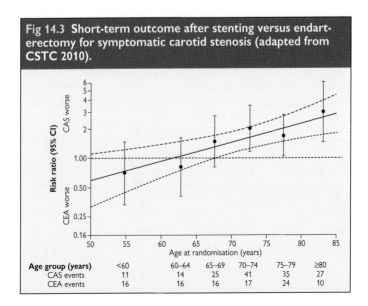

Fig 14.3 Short-term outcome after stenting versus endarterectomy for symptomatic carotid stenosis (adapted from CSTC 2010).

Age group (years)	<60	60–64	65–69	70–74	75–79	≥80
CAS events	11	14	25	41	35	27
CEA events	16	16	16	17	24	10

extracranial carotid stenosis. The risk of the composite primary outcome, which was different from that of earlier trials, included of stroke or death and myocardial infarction, did not differ significantly in the CAS group vs. the CEA group. However, the rate of stroke and death was still significantly higher in the CAS than in the CEA group, both during the periprocedural period and at 4 years (another important difference in study design when compared to earlier trials). During the periprocedural period, there was a higher risk of stroke with stenting and a higher risk of myocardial infarction with endarterectomy. The dilemma in the discussion about CREST results is the following question: are overall periprocedural stroke and MI equivalent complications with view to long-term outcome given the main goal for both procedures was to reduce the risk of stroke in patients with carotid disease (a low but long-term risk in asymptomatic subject and a moderate but short-term risk for symptomatic patients)? Although there may be some disagreement, patients (and experts) may think that this is not the case: in long-term views the effect of periprocedural MI was not significant, whereas the persistent disability after major and minor stroke on daily living and health conditions was obvious.

14.3.3 Intracranial and vertebral artery occlusive disease

14.3.3.1 Extracranial-intracranial anastomosis

Anastomosis between the extracranial and the intracranial arterial system (superficial temporal and middle cerebral arteries) is not beneficial in avoiding stroke in patients with stenosis or occlusion of middle cerebral artery (MCA) or internal carotid artery (ICA). Powers et al. recently re-investigated the hypothesis that EC-IC bypass surgery, added to best medical treatment, reduced stroke recurrences in patients with previous stroke from ICA occlusion. Despite using PET studies to recruit best suitable 195 candidates, who were randomized to receive surgery or not, the trial was terminated early for futility reasons: 2-year rates for primary endpoint were 21% (12.8%-29.2%, 95% CI) for the surgical vs. 22.7% (13.9-31.6%, 95% CI) for the non-surgical group (p=0.78).

14.3.4 Stenting of intracranial or vertebral artery stenosis

Patients with symptomatic intracranial stenoses higher than 50% are at significant risk of recurrent strokes, both in the anterior and posterior circulation. The incidence of complications after either angioplasty or stenting may be up to 6%. Several non-randomized trials have shown feasibility and acceptable safety of intracranial stenting, but the risk of restenosis remained high. Very recently the SAMMPRIS trial (Chimowitz et al. 2011) was stopped prematurely due to a high rate of early stroke after stenting. Therefore, aggressive medical treatment including adequate control of risk factors has been recommended in these patients. Also stenting of the extracranial segments

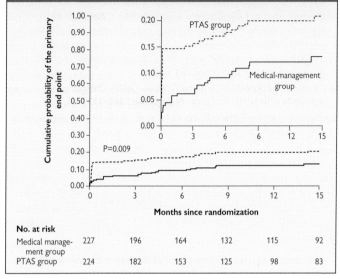

Fig 14.4 Kaplan–Meier curves for the cumulative probability of the primary end point, according to treatment assignment (adapted from Chimowitz et al. 2011).

of the vertebral artery is technical feasible with a moderate periprocedural risk, but there is a high rate of restenoses.

References

Adams HP, Jr, del Zoppo G, Alberts MJ, et. al. (2007) Guidelines for the early management of adults with ischaemic stroke: a guideline from the American Heart Association/American Stroke Association Stroke Council, Clinical Cardiology Council, Cardiovascular Radiology and Intervention Council, and the Atherosclerotic Peripheral Vascular Disease and Quality of Care Outcomes in Research Interdisciplinary Working Groups. *Stroke* **38**, 1655–711.

Amarenco P, Bogousslavsky J, Callahan A 3rd, Goldstein LB, Hennerici M, et al. (2006) High-dose atorvastatin after stroke or transient ischemic attack. *N Engl J Med* **355**(6), 549–59.

Bousser MG, Amarenco P, Chamorro A, Fischer M, et al. (2011) Terutroban versus aspirin in patients with cerebral ischaemic events (PERFORM): a randomised, double-blind, parallel-group trial. *Lancet* **377**(9782), 2013–22.

Brott TG, Hobson RW, Howard G, et al. (2010) Stenting versus Endarterectomy for Treatment of Carotid-Artery Stenosis. *N Engl J Med* **363**, 11–23.

Carotid Stenting Trialists' Collaboration (CSTC), Bonati LH, Dobson J, Algra A, et al. (2010) Short-term outcome after stenting versus endarterectomy for symptomatic carotid stenosis: a preplanned meta-analysis of individual patient data. *Lancet* **376**(9746), 1062–73.

Chimowitz MI, Lynn MJ, Derdeyn CP, et al. (2011) Stenting versus aggressive medical therapy for intracranial arterial stenosis. *N Engl J Med* **365**, 993–1003.

Conolly SJ, Eikelboom J, Joyner C, et al. (2011) Apixaban in patients with atrial fibrillation. *N Engl J Med* **364**, 806–17.

Connolly SJ, Ezekowitz MD, Yusuf S, et al. (2009) Dabigatran vs. warfarin inpatients with atrial fibrillation. *N Engl J Med* **361**, 1139–51.

Diener HC, Aichner F, Bode C, Böhm M, et al. (2010) Primary and secondary prevention of cerebral ischemia. Joint Guidelines of the German Society of Neurology (DGN) and German Stroke Society (DSG). *Akt Neurol* **37**, e2–e22.

European Stroke Organization (ESO) Executive Committee, ESO Writing Committee. (2008) Guidelines for management of ischaemic stroke and transient ischaemic attack 2008. *Cerebrovasc Dis* **25**, 457–507.

Furlan AJ, Reisman M, Massaro J, et al. (2012) Closure or medical therapy for cryptogenic stroke with patent foramen ovale. *N Engl J Med* **366**, 991–9.

Hankey JG, Eikelboom JW. (2010) Antithrombotic drugs for patients with ischaemic stroke and transient ischaemic attack to prevent recurrent major vascular events. *Lancet Neurol* **9**, 273–84.

Hankey JG. (2011) Hyperhomocystinaemia. *Cerebrovasc Dis* **32**(10), 603–7.

Granger CB, Alexander JH, McMurray JJ, et al.; ARISTOTLE Committees and Investigators. (2011) Apixaban versus warfarin in patients with atrial fibrillation. *N Engl J Med* **365**, 981–92.

Lincoff AM, Wolski K, Nicholls SJ, Nissen SE. (2007) Pioglitazone and risk of cardiovascular events in patients with type 2 diabetes mellitus: a meta-analysis of randomized trials. *JAMA* **298**(10), 1180–8.

Meier P, Knapp G, Tamhane U, Chaturvedi S, Gurm HS. (2010) Short term and intermediate term comparison of endarterectomy versus stenting for carotid artery stenosis: systematic review and meta-analysis of randomised controlled clinical trials. *BMJ* **340**:c467.

Patel MR, Mahaffey KW, Garg J, et al.; ROCKET AF Investigators. (2011) Rivaroxaban versus warfarin in nonvalvular atrial fibrillation. *N Engl J Med* **365**, 883–91.

Powers WJ, Clarke WR, Grubb RL, et al. (2011) Extracranial-intracranial bypass surgery for stroke prevention in hemodynamic cerebral ischemia. *JAMA* **306**, 1983–1992.

Rothwell, PM, Eliasziw M, Gutnikov SA, Warlow CP, Barnett HJ. Carotid Endarterectomy Trialists Collaboration. (2004) Endarterectomy for symptomatic carotid stenosis in relation to clinical subgroups and timing of surgery. *Lancet* **363**(9413), 915–24.

Szostak J, Laurant P. (2011) The forgotten face of regular physical exercise: a 'natural' anti-atherogenic activity. *Clin Sci (Lond)* **121**, 91–106.

Chapter 15

Recovery and rehabilitation

Key points

- The human brain has the unique ability to react adaptively to environmental changes, as well as to brain lesions. This ability is called cerebral plasticity.
- Neurorehabilitation is a multi-step process focusing on restoration or compensation of basal activities of daily living, and on psychosocial and community reintegration of the individual.
- Accordingly, future development of neurorehabilitation will be based on systematically evaluated methods, as well as on very individualized social reintegration.

15.1 Plasticity

The human brain shows a unique ability to react to changing internal (knowledge, learning, etc.) and external (environment) conditions leading to an appropriate adaptation. This permanent process is called plasticity. It can be demonstrated at organizational (synaptic sprouting), electrophysiological [long-term depression (LTD), long-term potentiation (LTP)], and macroscopic (changing of cortical networks) levels.

15.1.1 Plasticity after cerebral lesions

Focal brain lesions lead to direct loss of function, mediated by the affected neuronal assemblies. Beyond that, originally not affected corresponding areas may also be affected by the failure of the primary area. Within functional neuronal circuits focal lesions cause pathological disinhibition of corresponding areas via lack of inhibition leading to false up-regulation in the secondary areas or vice versa (lack of facilitation causing pathological inhibition in corresponding areas leading to false up-regulation).

Plasticity in focal injured brain can lead to recovery due to various mechanisms:

- Unmasking of previously 'hidden' control circuits
- Use of functional redundancy in different areas
- Vicariation, i.e. functional take-over by adjacent or remote areas.

Recovery can be achieved either by functional restoration or by compensation. Plasticity-driven compensation could be only partially successful or might be even counterproductive in the case of outflowing maladaptive plasticity (e.g. task-specific cranial dystonia, phantom pain).

15.2 **Neurorehabilitation**

Neurorehabilitation is a process aimed at supporting recovery after nervous system lesions. According to the multiple functions of the human brain, it addresses multiple domains (cognition, speech, motor, and sensory function). In addition to the rehabilitation process, it takes psychological, social cultural dimensions of the patient, and his family and environment into account. This complexity is mirrored in the International Classification of Functioning, Disability and Health (ICF) by the World Health Organization (WHO), a refined new classification of functioning and disability augmenting the International Classification of Diseases (ICD).

The ICF is structured in three levels:

- Health condition (ICD)
- Three central components:
  - Body functions and structure
  - Activities (by an individual) and participation (contribution in a life situation)
  - Additional information on severity and environmental factors
- Contextual factors (environmental factors, personal factors) (Figure 15.1).

Function and disability are considered as a dynamic interaction between the health of the individual and personal factors, as well as contextual factors of the environment. It allows a neutral description focusing on function, rather than condition or aetiology of a disease. It is relevant across cultures as well as for different ages, groups, and genders.

Neurorehabilitation is a multiple-step process focusing on restoration or compensation of basal activities of daily living (e.g. personal hygiene, dressing and undressing, eating, transferring from bed to chair and toilet, and back, voluntarily controlling urinary and bowel discharge, moving around). In addition, the process of rehabilitation

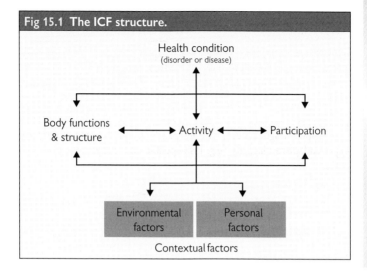

Fig 15.1 The ICF structure.

Health condition
(disorder or disease)

Body functions
& structure ⟷ Activity ⟷ Participation

Environmental
factors

Personal
factors

Contextual factors

is aimed at the re-integration of the individual within his/her spe-cific community (e.g. social, cultural, occupational). In order to cope with the new situation of impaired activity and participation due to a neurological disease affecting structure and function of the ner-vous system, the patient and his social environment have to establish a 'new way of living'. Therefore, neurorehabilitation can be con-ceived as a holistic, patient, and community-focused discipline. This approach needs a multidisciplinary team working together with the patient in a mutual co-operation and transdisciplinary interaction.

15.3 **Empiric treatment methods**

Traditional neurorehabilitation methods have been developed in the 1950s and 60s and refined in several rehabilitation 'schools' (e.g. Bobath, Perfetti, Vojta). Due to the highly variable functional deficits after lesions of the nervous system, many empirical methods have been proposed, used, and modified over the years. Because of the heterogeneous groups of patients and the difficulty of creating adequate control groups in sufficient number of cases, as well as the regrettably presence of dogmatic thinking, hardly any of these clas-sical methods were reviewed in systematic randomized clinical trials to proof their efficacy.

However, the lack of evidence-based treatment concepts should not provide arguments of overall ineffectiveness, as everyday reha-bilitation shows causative improvement in many patients, and better concepts have more recently been proposed and investigated.

15.4 **Evidence-based neurorehabilitation**

Fortunately, there are an increasing number of systematic trials evaluating classical, as well as new methods in neurorehabilitation, both in controlled small-sample trials and multicentre studies. However, a central problem is the definition of a specific, valid, and measurable endpoint. This is more easily possible for basal functions (defined simple movements series, e.g. Motricity Index, Fugl–Meyer test) than in complex endpoints (e.g. re-integration in social and occupational environment). Therefore, there are more and more well-designed controlled studies, concerning these basal functions (e.g. robot-assisted therapy in arm rehabilitation).

15.5 **Individualized neurorehabilitation**

Even more marked than in pharmacogenomics hitting for an individualized medicine analysis of genomic pattern with corresponding pharmacological responses in individual patient, neurorehabilitation needs a highly individualized customized approach for each individual patient according to the contextual factors as described in ICF. This very personalized method copes with the individualized situation of each patient, but method-implied generally valid endpoints are difficult to define in this approach.

15.6 **Specific neurorehabilitation**

In neurorehabilitation of motor deficits physiotherapists, as well as hand therapists treat the different pattern of motor dysfunction (paresis, spasticity, dystonia). Modern modular therapies are based on elementary knowledge about motor learning, such as repetition of elementary movement sequences, task-specific-training, and avoiding learned non-use. Fast specific training, feedback, and the extended activities of daily living, like transferring, walking, stair climbing, and mobility in domestic environment are, however, the subjects of rehabilitative therapy (Fig. 15.3 shows treadmill training as one typical example of rehabilitation procedures). Occupational therapists focus on re-integration in the individual or an adapted occupational environment in employed patients or in the restoration of age-based activities. Speech therapists attempt to improve verbal communication. They treat language disorders (aphasia, buccofacial apraxia, dyslexia, dyscalculia, dysgraphia), as well as dysarthria. Furthermore, they take care of dysphagia problems, which are often overlooked, but a very important element of neurological

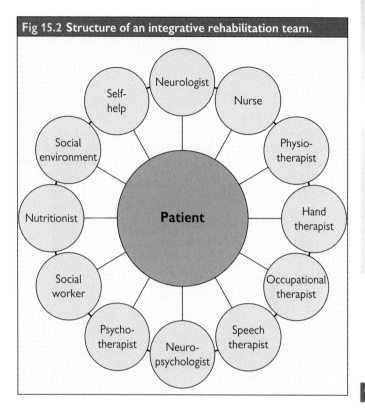

Fig 15.2 Structure of an integrative rehabilitation team.

Neurologist

Self-help

Nurse

Social environment

Physio-therapist

Nutritionist

Patient

Hand therapist

Social worker

Occupational therapist

Psycho-therapist

Neuro-psychologist

Speech therapist

disability. In cases of incomplete recovery, speech therapists also offer assistive technologies, such as an electronic voice box, or nutritional support by percutaneous endoscopic gastrostomy. Cognitive therapy is offered by clinical neuropsychologists, who treat the patient with sophisticated diagnosis by practical applications, as well as computer-assisted procedures.

The mission of an integrative rehabilitation team (Figure 15.2) including social workers is the psychosocial and community re-integration of the patient. This includes a return to the domestic environment, the organization of support by the welfare centre or transferring to a rest home, the re-integration into the previous occupational situation or in an adapted employment, and last, but not least, the resettlement of former social networks.

Fig 15.3 Example of a typical rehabilitation procedure.

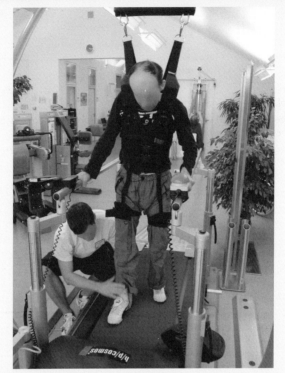

Treadmill training with partial body weight support in a patient with moderate right-sided hemiparesis and severe gait ataxia due to brainstem and cerebellar ischemia after basilar artery thrombosis

15.7 **Future development**

Future development of neurorehabilitation will lead into two directions:

- Increased use of knowledge from basic neuroscience for movement therapies (knowledge about motor learning by imitation and imagination, or robot-assisted therapies) augmented by neuromodulation tools (pharmaceutical agents, transcranial magnetic or direct current stimulation)
- Development of better psychosocial and community re-integration therapies, leading to a highly individualized rehabilitation therapy.

References

Alonso-Alonso M, Fregni F, Pascual-Leone A. (2007) Brain stimulation in poststroke rehabilitation. *Cerebrovasc Dis* **24**(Suppl 1), 157–66.

Bolognini N, Pascual-Leone A, Fregni F. (2009) Using non-invasive brain stimulation to augment motor training-induced plasticity. *J Neuroeng Rehabil* **6**, 8.

Dobkin BH. (2004) Neurobiology of rehabilitation. *Ann NY Acad Sci* **1038**, 148–70.

Hallett M. (2001) Plasticity of the human motor cortex and recovery from stroke. *Brain Res Brain Res Rev* **36**, 169–74.

Hömberg, V. (2005) Additive medicine in neurorehabilitation—a critical review. *Acta Neurochir* **93**, 3–14.

Kwakkel G, Kollen B, Lindeman E. (2004) Understanding the pattern of functional recovery after stroke: facts and theories. *Restor Neurol Neurosci* **22**, 281–99.

Langhorne P, Coupar F, Pollock A. (2009) Motor recovery after stroke: a systematic review. *Lancet Neurol* **8**, 741–54.

Lo AC, Guarino PD, Richards LG, et al. (2010) Robot-assisted therapy for long-term upper-limb impairment after stroke. *N Engl J Med* **362**, 1772–83.

Seitz RJ, Bütefisch CM, Kleiser R, Hömberg V. (2004) Reorganisation of therapial circuit in human brain disease. *Restor Knew Designs* **22**, 207–29.

Ward NS. (2004) Functional reorganization of the cerebral motor system after stroke. *Curr Opin Neurol* **17**, 725–30.

Index